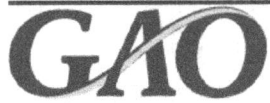

United States Government Accountability Office

Report to the Ranking Member, Committee on Finance, U.S. Senate

June 2013

MEDICAID DEMONSTRATION WAIVERS

Approval Process Raises Cost Concerns and Lacks Transparency

GAO-13-384

GAO Highlights

Highlights of GAO-13-384, a report to the Ranking Member, Committee on Finance, U.S. Senate

June 2013

MEDICAID DEMONSTRATION WAIVERS
Approval Process Raises Cost Concerns and Lacks Transparency

Why GAO Did This Study

Medicaid, a $436 billion federal and state health care program for low-income individuals and families, is a significant and growing expenditure. Section 1115 of the Social Security Act authorizes the Secretary of Health and Human Services to waive certain Medicaid requirements and allow otherwise uncovered costs for demonstration projects that are likely to promote Medicaid objectives. By HHS policy, these demonstrations should be budget neutral, that is, not increase federal spending over what it would have been if the state's existing program had continued. States estimate what their spending would have been without the demonstration, and HHS approves a spending based on projected spending.

GAO was asked to review HHS approval of recent Medicaid section 1115 demonstrations. GAO examined (1) the purpose of new demonstrations, and (2) the extent to which HHS's policy and process for reviewing proposed demonstration spending provide assurances that federal costs will not increase. For 10 new comprehensive demonstrations approved from January 2007 through May 2012, GAO reviewed application, approval, and budget neutrality documents provided by HHS; calculated estimated spending limits; and interviewed HHS officials.

What GAO Recommends

GAO recommends that HHS update its budget neutrality policy and reexamine spending limits for the Arizona and Texas demonstrations. HHS disagreed with GAO's recommendations. GAO believes these steps are needed to improve the budget neutrality process.

View GAO-13-384. For more information, contact Katherine Iritani at (202) 512-7114 or iritank@gao.gov.

What GAO Found

The 10 new demonstrations GAO examined expanded states' use of federal funds and implemented new coverage strategies. Arizona and Texas established funding pools to make new supplemental payments beyond what they could have made under traditional Medicaid requirements and receive federal matching funds for the payments. All 10 demonstrations were approved to use different coverage strategies or impose new cost sharing requirements, including limiting benefits or imposing deductibles for certain populations.

The Department of Health and Human Services' (HHS) budget neutrality policy and process did not provide assurances that all recently approved demonstrations will be budget neutral. For 4 of 10 demonstrations GAO reviewed, HHS approved spending limits that were based on assumptions of cost growth that were higher than its benchmark rates, and that, in some cases, included costs states never incurred in their base year spending. HHS's benchmark growth rates are the lower of the state's recent growth rates or projections for Medicaid program growth nationwide. For example, HHS approved a spending limit for Arizona's demonstration using outdated information on spending—1982 data that was projected forward—that reflected significantly higher spending than what the state's Medicaid program had actually cost. For Texas, HHS approved a spending limit using a base year that included billions in costs the state had not incurred. GAO found limited support and documentation for the higher-than-benchmark limits HHS approved. If HHS had held the 4 demonstrations' spending to levels suggested by its policy, the 5-year spending limits would have been an estimated $32 billion lower than what was approved; the estimated federal share of this reduction would be about $21 billion.

Comparison of 5-Year Medicaid Spending Limits as Approved by the Department of Health and Human Services (HHS) and as Estimated Using Benchmark Growth Rates and Actual Costs for Selected Demonstrations Approved between January 2007 and May 2012

Dollars in millions, federal and state spending

State	HHS-approved	GAO estimate using benchmark growth rates and actual costs	Difference
Arizona	$72,679	$46,382	$26,297
Indiana	10,626	10,211	416
Rhode Island	12,075	11,303	772
Texas	142,394	137,987	4,567
Total	$237,774	$205,723	$32,051

Source: GAO analysis of HHS data.

For 6 other demonstrations, the approved spending limits reflected the states' actual historical costs or criteria that were specified in law, which HHS followed. In examining HHS's current written budget neutrality policy, GAO found that the policy is outdated and does not include a process for assuring the reliability of the data used to set spending limits. GAO has previously suggested that Congress require HHS to improve its budget neutrality process, in part, by improving the review criteria and methods, and by documenting and making clear the basis for approved limits. In addition to these suggestions, GAO believes HHS needs to take further actions to address the findings in this report.

United States Government Accountability Office

Contents

Letter		1
	Background	5
	New Demonstrations Allowed States to Change How They Used Federal Funds, and to Implement New Coverage Strategies	11
	For 4 of 10 Reviewed Demonstrations, HHS's Policy and Process for Approving Spending Limits Did Not Provide Assurances That Demonstrations Will Not Increase Federal Costs	22
	Conclusions	32
	Recommendations for Executive Action	33
	Agency Comments and Our Evaluation	33
Appendix I	Summary of Submitted and Reviewed Applications for Comprehensive Section 1115 Medicaid Demonstrations	36
Appendix II	A Summary of Key Features of Recent Demonstrations	40
Appendix III	Comments from the Department of Health and Human Services	48
Appendix IV	GAO Contact and Staff Acknowledgments	53
Related GAO Products		54

Tables

Table 1: Comparison of 5-Year Medicaid Spending Limits Approved by the Department of Health and Human Services (HHS) and Estimated Spending Limits Using Benchmark Growth Rates and Actual Costs   23

Table 2: Comparison of Growth Rates Approved by the Department of Health and Human Services (HHS) for the Arizona Medicaid Demonstration and Benchmark Growth Rates   25

Table 3: Comparison of Growth Rates Approved by the Department of Health and Human Services (HHS) for the Indiana Medicaid Demonstration and Benchmark Growth Rates	27
Table 4: National and State-Historical Growth Rates that the Department of Health and Human Services (HHS) Compared in Selecting a Base Year and Approving the Rhode Island Medicaid Demonstration	27
Table 5: Status of Comprehensive Section 1115 Medicaid Demonstration Applications, by State, Submitted to the Department of Health and Human Services (HHS) from January 2007 through May 2012	37

Figure

Figure 1: Overview of the Department of Health and Human Services' (HHS) Process for Projecting the Future Cost of a State's Existing Medicaid Program	10

Abbreviations

CHIP	State Children's Health Insurance Program
CHIPRA	Children's Health Insurance Program Reauthorization Act of 2009
CMS	Centers for Medicare & Medicaid Services
DSH	Disproportionate Share Hospital
DSRIP	Delivery System Reform Incentive Payment
FMAP	Federal Medical Assistance Percentage
FPL	federal poverty level
HHS	Department of Health and Human Services
HIP	Healthy Indiana Plan
OMB	Office of Management and Budget
PPACA	Patient Protection and Affordable Care Act
SNCP	Safety Net Care Pool
UC	Uncompensated Care
UPL	Upper Payment Limit

This is a work of the U.S. government and is not subject to copyright protection in the United States. The published product may be reproduced and distributed in its entirety without further permission from GAO. However, because this work may contain copyrighted images or other material, permission from the copyright holder may be necessary if you wish to reproduce this material separately.

GAO
U.S. GOVERNMENT ACCOUNTABILITY OFFICE

441 G St. N.W.
Washington, DC 20548

June 25, 2013

The Honorable Orrin G. Hatch
Ranking Member
Committee on Finance
United States Senate

Dear Senator Hatch:

The Medicaid program—a $436 billion joint federal-state program that finances health care coverage for low-income populations, including children and aged or disabled adults—involves significant and growing expenditures for the federal government and states. Under section 1115 of the Social Security Act, the Secretary of Health and Human Services may waive certain federal Medicaid requirements and allow costs that would not otherwise be covered for experimental, pilot, or demonstration projects that are likely to promote Medicaid objectives.[1] These demonstrations also allow states to test and evaluate new approaches for delivering Medicaid services.[2] In fiscal year 2011, $57.5 billion in federal funds, or about one-fifth of the $260 billion in federal Medicaid expenditures, were for services, coverage initiatives, and delivery system redesigns provided under section 1115 demonstrations in 40 states. For 10 of these states, more than half of their total federal Medicaid expenditures were for section 1115 demonstrations.

Under Department of Health and Human Services (HHS) policy, section 1115 demonstrations should not be approved unless they are budget neutral to the federal government; that is, the federal government will spend no more under a state's demonstration than it would have spent

---

[1] 42 U.S.C. § 1315(a). In this report, we refer to these Medicaid demonstrations as "section 1115 demonstrations" or "demonstrations."

[2] Although the Secretary of Health and Human Services has delegated the administration of the Medicaid program, including the approval of section 1115 demonstrations, to the Centers for Medicare & Medicaid Services (CMS), we refer to HHS throughout this report because section 1115 demonstration authority ultimately resides with the Secretary. Other HHS offices and agencies may be involved in the review and approval of these demonstrations.

without the demonstration.[3] Budget neutrality generally is not a statutory requirement; however, HHS's policy requires states to show that their demonstrations will be budget neutral as part of their application to HHS. Once approved, each demonstration operates under a negotiated budget neutrality agreement that places a limit on federal Medicaid spending over the life of the demonstration. In assessing a state's projected spending limit, HHS's policy calls for using estimates of growth that are the lower of: (1) the state's historical growth for Medicaid in recent years, or (2) the President's budget Medicaid trend rate projected for the nation. The lower rate is referred to as the benchmark growth rate.[4]

We have had long-standing concerns with HHS's policy, process, and criteria for reviewing and approving section 1115 demonstrations, including the absence of a federal process for obtaining public input and a lack of transparency in the basis for approved spending limits.[5] For example, we previously found that although some demonstrations had the potential to significantly affect beneficiaries, advocates and others had not had an opportunity to review and provide input prior to the demonstrations' approval. In recent years, Congress and HHS, however, have taken significant steps to improve the review and approval process, by establishing a public input process at the federal level before

---

[3]HHS has implemented a budget neutrality policy for section 1115 demonstrations since the 1980's. The most recent version of this policy was published in 2001. In this report, we refer to this budget neutrality policy as "HHS's policy."

[4]In this report we refer to the President's budget Medicaid trend rate as the national growth rate.

[5]GAO, *Medicaid Section 1115 Waivers: Flexible Approach to Approving Demonstrations Could Increase Federal Costs*, GAO/HEHS-96-44 (Washington, D.C.: Nov. 8, 1995); *Medicaid and SCHIP: Recent HHS Approvals of Demonstration Waiver Projects Raise Concerns*, GAO-02-817 (Washington, D.C.: July 12, 2002); *Medicaid Waivers: HHS Approvals of Pharmacy Plus Demonstrations Continue to Raise Cost and Oversight Concerns*, GAO-04-480 (Washington, D.C.: June 30, 2004); *Medicaid Demonstration Waivers: Lack of Opportunity for Public Input during Federal Approval Process Still a Concern*, GAO-07-694R (Washington, D.C.: July 24, 2007); *Medicaid Demonstration Waivers: Recent HHS Approvals Continue to Raise Cost and Oversight Concerns*, GAO-08-87 (Washington, D.C.: Jan. 31, 2008). Since 2003 Medicaid has been on our list of high-risk programs in part because of concerns about inadequate fiscal oversight, including oversight of section 1115 demonstrations. A list of related GAO reports appears at the end of this report.

demonstrations are approved.[6] We have also reported that HHS had approved spending limits that included impermissible costs in the baselines, that included hypothetical costs in the baselines, or that exceeded benchmark growth rates. As a result of these findings, we made recommendations to HHS in 2002 and 2004 to take certain steps to improve the budget neutrality process, such as (1) clarifying the criteria for reviewing and approving states' demonstration spending limits, (2) better ensuring that valid methods are used to demonstrate budget neutrality, and (3) documenting material explaining the basis for any approvals and making the material public.[7] In a 2008 report, because HHS disagreed with these recommendations, we suggested that Congress consider requiring that HHS take these actions to improve the section 1115 demonstration review process.[8] These issues, however, have not yet been addressed.

You expressed interest in the section 1115 demonstrations approved by HHS since we last reviewed selected demonstrations, which were approved from July 2004 through December 2006.[9] For this report, we reviewed a selection of new comprehensive section 1115 demonstration proposals approved since 2007 for (1) the purpose of the demonstrations, and (2) the extent to which HHS's policy and process for reviewing proposed spending under the demonstrations provides assurances that federal costs will not increase.

To describe the purpose of new comprehensive demonstrations HHS has approved since 2007, we reviewed all those approved from January 2007 through May 2012 and that were still operating in May 2012. We excluded demonstrations that were extensions and amendments of previously approved demonstrations and those that were not comprehensive, that is,

---

[6] The Patient Protection and Affordable Care Act (PPACA) required the Secretary of Health and Human Services to issue regulations for section 1115 applications and extensions that address certain topics including a state and federal public notice and comment process, submission of reports on implementation by states and periodic evaluation by HHS. In response, on February 27, 2012, HHS published final regulations establishing these requirements for new section 1115 Medicaid demonstration applications and extensions. Pub. L. No. 111-148, § 10201, 124 Stat.119, 922 (2010); 77 Fed. Reg. 11,678 (Feb. 27, 2012).

[7] GAO-02-817, GAO-04-480.

[8] GAO-08-87.

[9] GAO-08-87.

they were limited to one category of services. We also excluded demonstrations that extended coverage to new populations in response to Medicaid expansion, which can begin in 2014 under the Patient Protection and Affordable Care Act (PPACA).[10] We identified demonstrations submitted by 10 states that met these criteria: Arizona, the District of Columbia, Idaho, Indiana, Michigan, Missouri, New Mexico, Rhode Island, Texas, and Wisconsin.[11] We reviewed application and approval documents for each demonstration, and interviewed HHS officials.[12] We used certain characteristics to describe the purpose of the demonstrations, such as whether the demonstrations changed how the states used federal funds, expanded Medicaid coverage to a new population of beneficiaries, and implemented new cost sharing requirements.

To assess the extent to which HHS's policy and process provides assurances that federal costs will not increase over what they would have been in the absence of the demonstration, we reviewed HHS's policy. We also reviewed the documentation for the 10 new comprehensive demonstrations selected for the first objective and budget neutrality analyses prepared by the states and submitted to HHS. We examined the basis of HHS's approved federal and state combined spending limit for each demonstration, and determined whether HHS followed its policy for determining budget neutrality. We then compared the spending limits approved by HHS with our estimates of the spending limits. We calculated our estimate of the spending limits in accordance with HHS's policy by using the most recent year of expenditures provided by the state

---

[10]PPACA provides for the expansion of Medicaid eligibility to nonelderly individuals whose household income does not exceed 133 percent of the federal poverty level (FPL). PPACA also imposes a 5 percent income disregard when calculating modified adjusted gross income for determining Medicaid eligibility, which effectively increases this income level to 138 percent of the FPL for this population. Pub. L. No. 111-148, §§ 2001(a)(1), 2002(a), 124 Stat. 119, 271, 279, as amended by Pub. L. No. 111-152, § 1004(e), 124 Stat. 1029, 1034 (2010). This expansion is estimated to result in the enrollment of an additional 7 million individuals in 2014. Accordingly, beginning in 2014, states may provide coverage of these adults under their state plan as opposed to under a section 1115 demonstration.

[11]In this report, we use the term "state" to refer to the 50 states and the District of Columbia.

[12]We did not review the implementation of these demonstrations after they were approved. In addition, we reviewed documentation related to amendments, when necessary.

for the base year, and the lower of either the state's historical average cost growth rate or the estimate of the Medicaid national growth rate developed by the Centers for Medicare & Medicaid Services (CMS) actuary. We then estimated the federal share of the spending limits using the 2012 Federal Medical Assistance Percentage (FMAP) for each state.[13] In our assessment, we did not trace the underlying spending and enrollment data used to develop spending limits to source documentation on spending or determine whether the baseline expenditures included impermissible costs. To the extent baseline spending or enrollment were overstated or understated, our estimates of benchmark spending limits could also be overstated or understated. We determined that the data were sufficiently reliable for the purpose of examining the information that HHS used in making its decisions about budget neutrality. To supplement our reviews, we interviewed HHS and Office of Management and Budget (OMB) officials about HHS's policy and process for setting spending limits for demonstrations, the basis of the spending limits for the 10 demonstrations, and the steps taken to ensure the quality of the data used to set spending limits. We did not obtain documentation from state officials or discuss demonstration proposals, approvals, and cost data with state officials.

We conducted this performance audit from June 2012 to June 2013 in accordance with generally accepted government auditing standards. Those standards require that we plan and perform the audit to obtain sufficient, appropriate evidence to provide a reasonable basis for our findings and conclusions based on our audit objectives. We believe that the evidence obtained provides a reasonable basis for our findings and conclusions based on our audit objectives.

Background

Each state administers its Medicaid program in accordance with its own Medicaid plan, which determines the groups of individuals to be covered, services to be provided, methodologies for providers to be reimbursed, and the administrative requirements that states must meet. To receive federal matching dollars for services provided to Medicaid beneficiaries, each state must submit a Medicaid plan for review and approval by HHS. States must meet certain federal requirements, but have flexibility beyond

---

[13]The federal government matches state Medicaid expenditures for most services according to the state's FMAP. A state's FMAP is calculated using a statutory formula based on the state's per capita income in relation to the national per capita income.

these federal parameters. For example, states must cover certain "mandatory" populations and benefits, but they have the option of covering "optional" categories of individuals and benefits. Coverage of optional populations and benefits varies across the states.[14] States may also choose from different delivery systems, such as fee-for-service or managed care.[15]

States pay health care providers for covered services provided to Medicaid beneficiaries based on provider claims for services rendered. States generally make two types of supplemental payments to certain providers—payments separate from and in addition to those made to providers using regular Medicaid payment rates. Under federal law, states are required to make Disproportionate Share Hospital (DSH) payments to hospitals that serve a disproportionate share of low-income and Medicaid patients, in addition to regular Medicaid payments. Hospitals are subject to an annual limit on DSH payments, defined as the hospitals' uncompensated care costs for Medicaid and uninsured patients minus Medicaid payments, and payments made on behalf of uninsured patients.[16] States also make other supplemental payments, which are often referred to as non-DSH supplemental payments or "Upper Payment Limit (UPL) payments" to providers such as hospitals and nursing homes. These payments are based on the difference between Medicaid payments for services using regular Medicaid payment rates and the UPL, which is the ceiling on federal reimbursement.[17] In general, the use

---

[14]Nationally in 2007, optional populations accounted for about 30 percent of Medicaid enrollment and about 42 percent of all Medicaid spending in 2007; optional services accounted for about 33 percent of Medicaid expenditures.

[15]Under a Medicaid managed care program, states contract with managed care organizations, to provide or arrange for medical services, and prospectively pay the plans a fixed monthly rate, or capitation payment, per enrollee. States receive federal reimbursement for capitation payments and the plans pay providers, such as hospitals and physicians, for services provided to Medicaid enrollees.

[16]42 U.S.C. § 1396r-4. In addition, under federal law, states may only claim federal matching funds for DSH payments made to qualifying hospitals up to the states' DSH allotments. DSH allotments are based on a statutory formula and allotment amounts vary across the states.

[17]The UPL is based on a reasonable estimate of what Medicare—the federal health program that covers individuals aged 65 and over, individuals with end-stage renal disease, and certain disabled individuals—would pay for similar services. In addition, under UPL arrangements, payments are subject to aggregate limits by provider type, but there are not firm dollar limits on individual providers. See, for example, 42 C.F.R. §§ 447.272, 447.321.

of managed care to deliver Medicaid services precludes states from making UPL payments to providers because states are prohibited from making such payments for services provided under a managed care contract.[18]

Medicaid Section 1115 Demonstrations

Generally, the authority provided to the Secretary of Health and Human Services by section 1115 of the Social Security Act allows states to expand Medicaid coverage through demonstration projects to "expansion" populations that would not otherwise be eligible under traditional Medicaid programs. These demonstrations provide a way for states to innovate outside of many of Medicaid's otherwise applicable requirements. For example, states may test ways to obtain savings or efficiencies in how they deliver services in order to cover expansion populations. Under a demonstration, states may also alter their Medicaid benefit package for categories of covered populations. Without this authority, states generally would be required to provide covered benefits in the same amount, duration, and scope to all beneficiaries covered under the state plan.

States may have more than one comprehensive demonstration. For example, New Jersey had one demonstration targeted at expanding coverage to uninsured childless adults, and a separate demonstration targeted at expanding coverage to uninsured parents of Medicaid-eligible children. Both these demonstrations are comprehensive because they provide a broad range of services to these populations. States may also administer a large portion of their Medicaid program under a demonstration. For example, in Vermont, nearly all of the state's Medicaid expenditures in fiscal year 2011 were for costs associated with a demonstration.

Generally, to extend Medicaid to any previously uncovered populations or receive federal Medicaid matching funds for otherwise unallowable costs under the terms of a section 1115 demonstration, states must establish that the demonstration is budget neutral. To do so, states must show that their plans for changing their Medicaid program will generate savings to

---

[18]Federal regulations prohibit payments by a state Medicaid agency to providers for services rendered under a contract with managed care organizations, with the exception of DSH and graduate medical education payments. This prohibition extends to UPL payments. See 42 C.F.R. § 438.60.

Medicaid, or they must get approval for redirecting existing Medicaid funding to cover the expected costs of the demonstration. For example:

- States have expanded the population eligible for Medicaid coverage by implementing managed care. In these demonstrations, states established budget neutrality by showing they would achieve savings from enrollment in managed care that could be used to cover new populations under the demonstration.

- States also have been approved by HHS to redirect certain categories of federal Medicaid funding for new purposes under the demonstration. Specifically, states have received approval to use all or a portion of their DSH allotments to cover previously ineligible individuals and costs under their demonstrations.

- States also have expanded coverage to previously ineligible populations, but in order to maintain budget neutrality, have provided the expansion population with a reduced benefit package—such as not covering inpatient hospital care—as compared to the typical benefits provided to Medicaid beneficiaries. Other strategies have included imposing higher cost-sharing on services or capping enrollment for expansion populations.

Review Responsibilities for Demonstrations

States submit applications for section 1115 demonstrations to HHS. If HHS approves the demonstration, it is typically approved for a 5-year period.[19] States that want to renew an existing demonstration have the option of requesting an extension or submitting an application for a new demonstration. States that submit an application for a new demonstration instead of an extension would need to terminate the existing demonstration, and would be required to notify beneficiaries of potential changes in coverage. A federal review team examines applications for both new demonstrations and extensions. The review team is led by CMS

---

[19]As referenced above, in February 2012, HHS published a final rule that imposed new requirements for states seeking approval for section 1115 demonstrations. In implementing some of these requirements, in October 2012, HHS made available an interim template that states may use in submitting their applications for section 1115 demonstrations. The application requirements are slightly different for new applications than for extensions. For example, applications for extensions must report evidence of how the objectives of the prior demonstration have or have not been met and must include an evaluation report with findings to date.

and includes representatives from OMB; from other agencies within HHS as applicable, such as the Substance Abuse and Mental Health Services Administration providing a review of waivers that affect mental health; and HHS Secretarial offices including the Assistant Secretary for Planning and Evaluation and the Assistant Secretary for Financial Resources. CMS's Office of the Actuary provides nationwide data on projected Medicaid cost growth, but is not part of the federal review team. The federal review may consist of negotiations, including the exchange of questions and answers between the review team and the state. In approving applications, HHS might not approve all components of the states' request contained in their applications. (See app. I for a discussion of applications that were submitted and reviewed between January 2007 and May 2012.)

Determining Budget Neutrality for Demonstrations

According to HHS's policy, spending limits are based on the projected cost of continuing states' existing Medicaid programs without a demonstration. The higher the projected costs, the more federal funding states are eligible to receive. The spending limits can be either an annual per person limit or an aggregate spending limit that remains fixed for the entire length of the demonstration, or a combination of both. HHS policy states that demonstration spending limits will be calculated from two components:

- **Spending base**. States select a recently completed year that establishes base levels of expenditures for populations included in the proposed demonstration—a state's "spending base." States also identify beneficiary groups for inclusion in the proposed demonstration. For example, demonstrations may include beneficiary groups, such as aged, blind and disabled, or families with children. However, the spending base must exclude certain base year expenditures, such as impermissible provider payments.

- **Growth rates**. States should submit to HHS 5 years of historical data for per person costs and beneficiary enrollment in their existing Medicaid program. HHS's policy states that spending limits should be based on a benchmark growth rate, which is the lower of state-specific historical growth or the estimates of nationwide growth for the beneficiary groups included in the demonstration.[20] The policy

---

[20]HHS's policy is specific to per person cost growth rates and does not explicitly address the application of enrollment growth rates; however, HHS considers state historical and nationwide enrollment growth rates in establishing spending limits.

indicates that states, in providing HHS with state-specific historical growth rates, must also provide quantified explanations of any unusual changes in the trends. Nationwide projections of cost growth are developed by CMS actuaries to assist OMB in preparing the President's budget. Growth rates for determining budget neutrality can vary for different eligibility groups. For example, the nationwide estimates of per capita cost growth in Medicaid for fiscal year 2012 were 6.0 percent for children, 3.4 percent for aged individuals, 2.6 percent for blind and disabled individuals, and 2.5 percent for adults.

Figure 1 illustrates steps used to set spending limits for proposed section 1115 demonstrations.

Figure 1: Overview of the Department of Health and Human Services' (HHS) Process for Projecting the Future Cost of a State's Existing Medicaid Program

Establish spending base	Establish per person cost growth rates	Apply growth rates to base year and establish spending limits
• Select a recent (base) year to establish a spending base for making projections • Identify beneficiaries and programs that will be covered by the demonstration's terms and conditions[a] • Determine costs associated with these beneficiaries and programs in the base year	• **State-specific growth rate**: based on beneficiary cost and enrollment data from a 5-year historical period compared to • **Nationwide growth rate**: based on estimates of beneficiary cost and enrollment growth nationwide used to develop the President's budget • HHS guidelines call for selecting the lower of the two growth rates	• Establish total projected costs of the existing Medicaid program by multiplying spending base by per person cost growth rates for each of 5 years proposed for the demonstration • Set spending limits for demonstration based on total projected costs of existing Medicaid program for populations included in the demonstration

Source: GAO analysis of HHS information.

[a]For example, a state may propose, that certain groups of beneficiaries, such as aged and disabled beneficiaries, will operate under the terms of the state's approved state Medicaid plan rather than under the terms of the demonstration.

Some types of section 1115 demonstrations are not required to follow this process for determining spending limits. Specifically, for demonstrations that redirect a state's federal DSH funding, HHS policy is to base the spending limit on the lower of the state's DSH allotment or actual DSH expenditures prior to the demonstration.[21] In addition, there is another group of recent section 1115 demonstrations pursuant to which federal law has defined how to calculate budget neutrality. Specifically, under the Children's Health Insurance Program Reauthorization Act of 2009 (CHIPRA), states with existing section 1115 demonstrations covering childless adults using State Children's Health Insurance Program (CHIP) funding were required to end these projects.[22] States, however, could apply and receive approval for new section 1115 demonstrations through which they could continue to cover childless adults using Medicaid funds. CHIPRA required that these new demonstrations be budget neutral, and required HHS to use a defined process of identifying the spending base and growth rates for demonstration spending limits.

New Demonstrations Allowed States to Change How They Used Federal Funds, and to Implement New Coverage Strategies

The 10 new comprehensive section 1115 demonstrations we examined focused on implementing ways of using federal funds to pay for services not typically covered under Medicaid. All 10 demonstrations were approved to implement different coverage strategies or cost sharing for certain beneficiary populations. Appendix II provides a brief summary of the key features of 10 demonstrations.

---

[21] DSH allotments are the maximum amount of federal DSH funding that is available for each state. They are based on a statutory formula, and allotment amounts vary across the states.

[22] CHIP is a joint federal state program to finance health coverage for children in families with income too high to qualify for Medicaid.

HHS's Approvals Allowed Two States to Establish Funding Pools to Make New Types of Supplemental Payments

Two states we reviewed—Arizona and Texas—obtained the authority under their section 1115 demonstrations to establish funding pools for purposes of making supplemental payments and to receive federal matching funds for these payments.

Arizona Health Care Cost Containment System

As approved, Arizona's section 1115 demonstration allows the state to make new types of supplemental payments to providers, and allowed the state to establish a funding pool from which these payments could be made. Arizona has operated a comprehensive section 1115 demonstration for many years, under which the majority of the Medicaid population is enrolled in managed care. Under its previous demonstration, the state made DSH payments to hospitals, but did not make UPL payments to its providers because the majority of services were provided under managed care contracts. UPL payments for services provided under managed care are generally prohibited under federal regulations. In March 2011, the state requested to terminate its existing section 1115 demonstration in order to limit coverage of certain adult populations.[23] Subsequently, the state received approval for a new demonstration that continued the existing managed care delivery system, granted the authority for the state to make new types of supplemental payments to providers through a Safety Net Care Pool (SNCP), and expanded coverage to certain populations.

Under the demonstration, the state obtained the authority to claim federal matching funds for new types of supplemental payments made to providers from SNCP. The state did not commit any state funds for these supplemental payments and instead relied on the contributions of eligible government entities for the nonfederal share of payments. According to HHS officials, because these supplemental payments were created under the authority of the demonstration, they were not subject to certain federal requirements that would otherwise apply. For example, officials reported that they did not consider these to be DSH payments and therefore the

---

[23]The state reported that due to budget constraints, it could not continue its program of providing coverage to certain adults. To end the coverage, the state had to terminate the demonstration under which the coverage was provided. The adults the state would no longer cover were those without dependent children with family income up to and including 100 percent of the FPL as well as adults with income in excess of 100 percent of the FPL who had qualifying healthcare costs that reduce their income to or below 40 percent of the FPL.

federal reimbursement for SNCP payments exceeds the maximum amount Arizona is allowed to receive under its DSH allotment.[24] They were not considered to be UPL payments and therefore could be made even when services were provided under a managed care contract. According to HHS officials, the terms and conditions of the demonstration defined requirements for these payments. For example, under the terms and conditions, as the SNCP payments were Medicaid payments, HHS required they be subject to certain requirements when made to DSH hospitals. Specifically, SNCP payments received for inpatient or outpatient hospital costs were required to be counted against each hospital's annual DSH payment limit.[25]

The terms and conditions of Arizona's demonstration also included other federal requirements and limits for the SNCP payments. Specifically:

- For each year of the demonstration, the state was allowed to make up to $332 million—total federal and nonfederal funds—in payments to hospitals, clinics, and other nonhospital providers that have high levels of uncompensated care for medical services provided to Medicaid eligible and uninsured individuals.[26] Demonstration requirements also limited these SNCP payments for individual providers' to their costs of delivering services to Medicaid and uninsured individuals,[27] and prohibited SNCP payments for nonemergency services provided to noncitizens who were not eligible for Medicaid.

---

[24]Arizona's DSH allotment was capped at about $101 million in 2011.

[25]Under federal law, hospitals that qualify for DSH payments are subject to hospital-specific limits, meaning hospitals have a calculated ceiling on the amount of DSH payments they may receive annually. Specifically, DSH payments to individual hospitals are limited to the hospital's uncompensated care costs for Medicaid and uninsured patients minus Medicaid payments and payments made by or on behalf of uninsured patients.

[26]The demonstration's terms and conditions identify 4 hospitals, 13 clinics, and 3 hospital-based physicians groups as eligible to receive SNCP payments.

[27]The terms and conditions of the demonstration state that for any provider receiving an SNCP payment, the total of Medicaid payments, DSH payments, SNCP payments, and any other payments the provider received for medical services delivered to Medicaid and uninsured individuals cannot exceed the actual cost of providing the services.

- In addition to the $332 million, the state was allowed, for the first 2 years of the demonstration, to make up to $20 million—total federal and nonfederal funds—in payments that were previously made under a state-funded health program. Specifically, the state was approved to make payments to hospital trauma centers, hospital emergency departments, and rural hospitals across the state for clinical, professional, and operational costs. These payments were intended to help hospitals manage their uncompensated care costs. Prior to the demonstration, these were entirely state-funded payments that Arizona voters approved in 2002.

Other features of Arizona's demonstration included expanding coverage to two groups of children: children with family income at or below 175 percent of the federal poverty level (FPL), who were not otherwise eligible for Medicaid; and children up to age 19 with incomes between 100 and 200 percent of the FPL, who had access to employer sponsored health care coverage, and were not otherwise eligible for Medicaid. Total funding—federal and nonfederal funds—available for expansion was capped at about $77 million each year by the demonstration. The state was also allowed to extend the length of Medicaid coverage for postpartum women from the typical 60 days to 24 months. The total cost allowed for this program—federal and nonfederal—was $20 million.

Texas Healthcare Transformation and Quality Improvement Demonstration

Two of the purposes of the Texas section 1115 demonstration were to allow the state to expand its use of managed care statewide, and to authorize new supplemental payments through two new funding pools. Prior to the demonstration, the state provided services to most of the state's Medicaid population on a fee-for-service basis. Under this system, hospitals provided services to Medicaid-covered individuals and then submitted bills to the state for reimbursement based on the state's regular Medicaid payment rates. In addition, the state made DSH payments and UPL payments for hospital services provided on a fee-for-service basis.

Under the demonstration, HHS approved two new types of supplemental payments to be distributed through two funding pools. In creating these pools, the state did not commit any state funds and instead relied on the contributions of eligible government entities for the nonfederal share of payments.[28] Under one pool, called the Uncompensated Care (UC) pool, the state could obtain federal matching funds on provider payments totaling up to $17.6 billion over the 5-year term of the demonstration.[29] Under the second pool, called the Delivery System Reform Incentive Payment (DSRIP) pool, the state could obtain federal matching funds on provider payments totaling up to $11.4 billion over the 5-year term of the demonstration. The demonstration significantly increased the amount of federal funding Texas could claim for the two new types of supplemental payments. For example, in fiscal year 2011—the year prior to the demonstration—the state claimed federal matching funds on about $2.6 billion in UPL payments. Under the demonstration, the state was authorized to receive federal matching funds on $4.2 billion in payments made in the first year of the demonstration and on $6.2 billion in payments made in each of the remaining 4 years of the demonstration.

HHS officials told us that because the UC pool payments were created under the demonstration, they were not DSH or UPL payments and therefore were not subject to the federal requirements that govern those payments. Thus, as with Arizona, these payments were in addition to, and not limited by, the maximum cap on federal matching that was provided to the state under its DSH allotment.[30] Officials told us the UC pool payments also were not considered to be UPL payments and could be made for services provided to individuals enrolled in managed care. According to HHS, the terms and conditions of the demonstration established requirements and limits for the UC pool payments. Among other things, the terms and conditions required that these payments be limited to individual providers' uncompensated costs of delivering services

---

[28] In order to qualify for these supplemental payments, providers needed to participate in a regional healthcare partnership that included local government entities or providers that could fund the nonfederal share of supplemental payments. These regional health care partnerships developed regional health plans that identified health care providers, community needs, and improvement projects to fund with supplemental payments.

[29] Payments made from the UC pool in the first year of the demonstration were transition payments to hospitals and physician groups that previously received UPL payments under the Medicaid state plan for claims during fiscal year 2011. This transition period ensures that those providers are eligible to receive the level of Medicaid funding they received in prior years from UPL payments as the state developed how it would distribute funds from this pool under the demonstration.

[30] Texas's DSH allotment was capped at about $957 million in 2011.

to Medicaid beneficiaries and uninsured individuals.[31] Further, as with Arizona, because the UC pool payments were Medicaid payments, the payments for inpatient or outpatient hospital costs were required to be counted against the amount of DSH payments that an individual hospital could receive. The terms and conditions also allowed the state to make these Medicaid supplemental payments to a variety of providers for serving Medicaid and uninsured individuals. These providers included physician-practice groups, government ambulance providers, government dental providers, and rural health providers with no public hospitals.

The terms and conditions also established requirements for the DSRIP pool. According to these, the DSRIP pool was established to provide incentive payments to hospitals related to infrastructure and health care redesign changes as Texas prepared for the increase in Medicaid enrollment that was expected under PPACA beginning in 2014. The state received approval to make payments related to four main areas: (1) infrastructure development, which included hiring more physicians and the use of electronic health records systems at the provider level; (2) program innovation and redesign, which included implementing strategies, such as reducing inappropriate use of the emergency room and patient center care models; (3) quality improvements, which included interventions to reduce and manage chronic disease; and (4) population-focused improvements, which included obtaining data to monitor changes in health status and measuring preventive health activities. Like the UC pool payments, HHS officials told us that these payments are not subject to federal requirements that would apply to DSH and UPL payments, and instead are governed solely by the terms and conditions of the demonstration.[32] However, unlike UC pool payments, DSRIP payments are incentive payments and not reimbursement for providing health care services. Consequently, HHS does not require these payments to be

---

[31]Although the level of federal funding for these new supplemental payments was significantly increased, the UC pool payments were held to a facility cost-based standard for reimbursement rather than the state's historic UPL program.

[32]According to the terms and conditions, the state could not receive federal funding for expenditures from the DSRIP pool until key milestones are met including: HHS's approval of the state's plan for and status of forming regional health care partnerships; identification of the public hospitals directing each of these partnerships; and development of a list of projects related to the four main areas noted above. In addition, incentive payments from the pool would be based on successful completion of HHS-approved metrics submitted by the regional healthcare partnerships related to the four areas.

counted against the amount of DSH payments a hospital could receive under its hospital specific DSH limit.

The DSRIP payments were approved by HHS under the expectation that the state would be expanding its Medicaid coverage under PPACA; however, since the demonstration's approval, the state has not confirmed that it intends to expand Medicaid to new populations allowed under PPACA. At the time Texas's demonstration was approved, PPACA required all states to expand Medicaid coverage to a new mandatory category of low-income individuals, and states were eligible to receive enhanced federal funding for this population beginning in January of 2014.[33] However, subsequent to this approval, the U.S. Supreme Court ruled that any state that chooses not to expand Medicaid coverage will not be subject to a penalty of losing Medicaid funding for the entire program, and instead will only forego the enhanced funding for that population, therefore making the expansion a choice for the states.[34] In June 2013, a state law was enacted that would prohibit the state Medicaid agency from expanding Medicaid coverage.[35] In general, HHS can withdraw authorities to claim federal funding for expenditures under demonstrations in certain circumstances, including if it determines that the approval no longer promotes the objectives of the Medicaid program. However, HHS officials stated that the delivery system improvements that will result from the DSRIP pool payments will benefit low-income and Medicaid populations, whether the state expands Medicaid or not. HHS does not plan to revisit the terms and conditions of the Texas demonstration as it relates to the DSRIP pool, even if the state does not expand Medicaid as provided under PPACA.

---

[33]States that failed to provide Medicaid coverage to mandatory population categories were subject to the potential penalty of losing federal funding for their Medicaid program.

[34]See *National Federation of Independent Business, et al., vs. Sebelius, Sec. of Health and Human Services, et al.*, 132 S. Ct. 2566 (U.S. June 28, 2012).

[35]Prior to this however, the Governor of Texas sent a letter to HHS in July 2012 stating that the state did not intend to expand Medicaid.

HHS Approvals Allowed Four States to Redirect DSH Funds Primarily to Expand Coverage to New Populations

Indiana, the District of Columbia, Wisconsin, and Missouri were allowed to redirect all or a portion of their federal DSH allotment, primarily to cover populations made eligible for Medicaid under the terms of the demonstration. Three of the states—Indiana, the District of Columbia, and Wisconsin—were approved to use at least some of their DSH allotment solely for coverage expansion.

- Indiana was allowed to use a portion of its DSH allotment to pay for services for a new population of about 36,000 higher-income parents and childless adults.[36]

- The District of Columbia demonstration expanded full Medicaid coverage to childless adults with incomes higher than the income level that would qualify them for Medicaid coverage under PPACA beginning in 2014—over 133 percent of the FPL. Individuals in this expansion population were previously covered under a local program for which the District of Columbia did not receive federal matching funds.[37]

- Wisconsin was approved to expand its plan to an estimated 35,000 childless adults, providing them with benefits, such as physician and hospital services.

The fourth state, Missouri, was also approved to redirect a portion of its DSH allotment for new purposes established under the demonstration, including, among other things, providing coverage to previously ineligible populations. Missouri was also allowed to redirect a portion of its DSH funds for payments for other purposes, as authorized under the demonstration, including

---

[36]These adults included uninsured adults who are custodial parents and caretakers of children eligible for Medicaid and CHIP. Also included were noncustodial parents or childless adults, ages 19 through 64 with family incomes up to and including 200 percent of the FPL who were not otherwise eligible for Medicaid or Medicare, who did not have access to an employer-sponsored health plan, had been uninsured for 6 months, and whose health care expenditures did not exceed a $1 million lifetime maximum on benefits under the demonstration. The demonstration also allowed the continued coverage of about 600,000 Medicaid enrollees.

[37]Under the previous program enrollees did not receive mental health and transportation benefits and they had a limited pharmacy network.

- payments to health clinics that provided ambulatory services to uninsured and indigent populations in and near St. Louis;[38]

- payments for administrative costs—nonhospital services—to a health commission, which will coordinate, monitor, submit reports on the demonstration's activities, and make recommendations for payment allocations;[39]

- a program that educated patients on primary care and proper use of the emergency room;[40] and

- the initiation of a coverage expansion pilot that would provide a limited primary care benefit package and test the use of a voucher system to provide acute hospital services when needed by individuals in the pilot expansion population.

HHS Approved a Global Cap for One State's Demonstration

Under the Rhode Island demonstration, HHS allowed a funding approach that established an overall spending—or global cap—on the federal matching funds for the state's Medicaid program. This cap puts the state at risk for any expenditures in excess of the cap, as the state is required to continue providing coverage for its Medicaid population using state funds. HHS gave the state new flexibility to manage its program by allowing Rhode Island to consolidate its Medicaid program under one comprehensive section 1115 demonstration, incorporating populations and services previously covered under the state plan, a previous section

---

[38]Prior to the demonstration, hospital systems in Missouri funded a system to pay for services provided to indigent individuals. For economic reasons, the hospitals stopped providing payments, and the state submitted its demonstration proposal in efforts to obtain federal matching funds for these payments.

[39]These costs—both state and federal—could not exceed $75,000 for 2 years of the demonstration or $300,000 for 3 years of the demonstration.

[40]This program worked with uninsured individuals that come to the emergency rooms and educated them on available resources for primary/non-emergent care, scheduled follow-up appointments with primary care providers, and arranged transportation to appointments. These services were coordinated while the individuals were in the emergency room. The costs—both state and federal—for this program could not exceed $175,000 per year for 2 years of the demonstration or $700,000 per year for 3 years.

1115 demonstration, and multiple other Medicaid waivers.[41] According to HHS, this consolidation would allow Rhode Island to seamlessly provide services to individuals who previously had to qualify to receive services, such as home and community-based services through different programs that were governed by different rules and authorities. The state's proposal indicated that this flexibility would allow the state to better manage the use of long-term care and increase home and community-based services. Through the demonstration, the state also was given the flexibility to make certain programmatic changes to its Medicaid program without having to follow more formal procedures. For example, for certain changes, such as those that would otherwise need to be processed as an amendment to the Medicaid state plan or to the demonstration terms and conditions or that did not affect eligibility or benefits, the state was allowed to only notify HHS of the change.[42] HHS officials noted that this was the first time they approved a test of this type of administrative flexibility.

HHS's Approvals Allowed Three States to Use Medicaid Funds to Continue Coverage to Expansion Populations

Idaho, Michigan, and New Mexico were required by federal law to discontinue using CHIP funds to cover childless adults, but were allowed to continue services for this population with Medicaid funds under a new section 1115 demonstration. These three states each applied and received approval for new demonstrations to continue to provide coverage to childless adults, without expanding to any new populations. Under these demonstrations, various types of benefits were provided to the childless adult populations. For example, Idaho was approved to provide premium assistance for qualifying employer-sponsored insurance, while Michigan and New Mexico were approved to provide coverage for services. Michigan was approved to limit benefits to outpatient services, and New Mexico was approved to provide coverage for both inpatient and outpatient services.

---

[41]Some of these populations were covered under a previous section 1915(c) waiver. Under a section 1915(c) waiver, states may provide coverage of services for a targeted population that may not otherwise be available under the state's Medicaid plan. Specifically, states may provide home or community-based health care to beneficiaries who would, if not for the services provided under the waiver, require institutional care.

[42]Under the demonstration, the state was required to categorize the types of changes it may make to the demonstration, and for certain categories the state was authorized to notify HHS of the change rather than submit an amendment to the Medicaid state plan or the demonstration.

States Were Approved to Implement Different Coverage Strategies and New Cost Sharing on Certain Populations through the Demonstrations

All 10 states we reviewed were approved to implement new ways of expanding coverage or imposing cost sharing requirements on different Medicaid populations. Examples of these strategies are presented below.

- Arizona's demonstration allowed, for a limited time, the state to charge expansion enrollees a fee when they miss a physician appointment in order to encourage proper use of medical services.[43] The demonstration also allowed the state to impose cost sharing for non-emergency use of the emergency room, as well as higher cost sharing for brand name drugs when a generic is available.[44]

- Indiana's demonstration allowed the state to establish a high-deductible health plan and health care spending account for uninsured adults enrolled for coverage under the demonstration. Expansion enrollees must make specified contributions to their accounts, based on income levels, as a condition of continued enrollment. The accounts must be used by enrollees to pay for the cost of health care services until a deductible is reached; however, preventive services up to a maximum amount would be exempt from this requirement. The spending account was intended to provide incentives for participants to utilize services in a cost-efficient manner. This demonstration also allowed the state to impose an enrollment cap on the number of childless adult expansion enrollees for its health savings account program.

- Three states—Idaho, Michigan, and New Mexico—were approved to continue some coverage strategies from their previous

---

[43] This fee was not applicable to those residing in two counties, and the application of the fee was at the provider's discretion.

[44] HHS's approval of this cost sharing, however, has been subject to legal challenges. On February 7, 2013, a court held that HHS's approval of this cost sharing for individuals only eligible under the demonstration was invalid. Specifically, the court determined that because HHS failed to consider expert opinions on the negative effects of cost sharing, the agency's decision to approve the cost sharing was arbitrary and capricious, in violation of the Administrative Procedure Act. The court required HHS to reevaluate this approval and develop a plan to address the deficiencies by May 2013. See Wood, et al. v. Betlach, et al., 2013 WL 474369 (D. Ariz. 2013). On April 8, 2013, the Secretary issued a new approval letter for Arizona, reaffirming the prior approval of increased cost sharing for certain segments of the demonstration population. In this letter HHS stated that, in light of the court's decision, HHS had reconsidered the state's request and had reanalyzed the administrative record, including objections raised by interested parties.

demonstrations.[45] For example, Idaho's premium assistance demonstration required a 50 percent employer contribution toward the cost of the health benefit plan. Michigan's demonstration allowed the state to continue to provide a limited benefit package that focused on outpatient services and required prior authorization for some of these services. Finally, New Mexico's demonstration allowed the state to cap medical expenditures for each enrollee.

- Rhode Island was allowed to form and pay for entities dedicated to reviewing the needs of enrollees eligible for long-term care. According to the state's proposal, this process facilitated the appropriate care setting by shifting care away from high-cost institutional settings when less costly home and community-based care was appropriate. The organization did this by helping enrollees decide how to manage their health care needs based on a distinction given to them as "highest need," "high need," or "preventive." This designation allowed the state to determine which cost-effective, long-term services an enrollee could receive. For example, those designated as highest need were approved to receive nursing home care, while those designated as preventive were approved to receive certain home health services.

For 4 of 10 Reviewed Demonstrations, HHS's Policy and Process for Approving Spending Limits Did Not Provide Assurances That Demonstrations Will Not Increase Federal Costs

For 4 of 10 demonstrations we reviewed, HHS approved spending limits that were based on assumptions of cost growth that were higher than those reflected by the state's historical spending and the President's budget. In addition, in some cases the approved spending limits included costs in the base year that were hypothetical. If HHS had held spending limits in the four demonstrations to levels suggested by its policy, we estimate that the spending limits would have been $32 billion lower over the 5-year term of the demonstrations. We also found that HHS's budget neutrality policy is out-dated, because it does not reflect HHS's current processes or provide assurances that data used for spending limits are reliable.

---

[45]These states were required by federal law to discontinue using CHIP funds to cover childless adults, but were allowed to continue services for this population with Medicaid funds under a new section 1115 demonstration.

HHS Approved Spending Limits for Four States Based on Growth Projections That Exceeded Benchmarks and Included Hypothetical Costs, with Limited Support

HHS approved spending limits for the Arizona, Indiana, and Rhode Island demonstrations that used growth rates that exceeded benchmark rates and, in the case of Texas, included hypothetical costs in the base year spending. HHS officials reported that their policy and process allow for negotiations in determining spending limits, including adjustments to the benchmark policy. However, HHS's policy does not specify criteria and methods for such adjustments or the documentation and support needed for adjustments. We found that the criteria and methods for making the adjustments in these states were not always clear or well supported. Our estimates show that, had HHS used benchmark growth rates and actual base year costs, the 5-year spending limits would have been almost $32 billion dollars lower than what was actually approved. The federal share of the $32 billion reduction would constitute an estimated $21 billion. (See table 1.)

Table 1: Comparison of 5-Year Medicaid Spending Limits Approved by the Department of Health and Human Services (HHS) and Estimated Spending Limits Using Benchmark Growth Rates and Actual Costs

Dollars in millions

State	HHS-approved spending limit	Estimate of spending limit using benchmark growth rates and actual base year costs	Increase in spending in HHS approved spending limit	Estimated federal share of increase in spending limit[a]
Arizona[b]	$72,679	$46,382	$26,297	17,698
Indiana	10,626	10,211	416	278
Rhode Island	12,075	11,303	772	402
Texas	142,394	137,827	4,567	2,659
Total	**$237,774**	**$205,723**	**$32,051**	**$21,037**

Source: GAO analysis of HHS data.

Notes: These demonstrations were approved between January 2007 and May 2012. Spending limits approved by HHS and our estimates of spending limits under HHS's policy reflect limits on total federal and state spending. We calculated spending limits under HHS's policy using the most recent year of expenditures provided by the state for the base year and benchmark growth rates, that is, the lower of either the state's historical average cost growth rate or the estimate of Medicaid cost growth nationwide provided by the Centers for Medicare & Medicaid Services' (CMS) actuary. We also excluded hypothetical costs. Column totals may not add due to rounding.

[a]The estimated federal share is based on the 2012 Federal Medical Assistance Percentage (FMAP) for each of the four states. The federal government matches state Medicaid expenditures for most services according to the state's FMAP. A state's FMAP is calculated using a statutory formula based on the state's per capita income in relation to the national per capita income.

[b]Amounts represent the spending limit for four of the six beneficiary groups included in the demonstration. For the remaining two groups, HHS's documentation did not include historical enrollment because they were new populations covered under the demonstration and no enrollment data existed. As a result, we could not calculate a spending limit for them. This figure also does not

reflect other components of the demonstration's total spending limit, including a maximum of about $1.8 billion for supplemental payments to finance uncompensated care and other activities.

Arizona

HHS departed from its policy in selecting base year expenditures and benchmark growth rates for the approved Arizona spending limit without a clear rationale. Had actual base year expenditures and benchmark growth rates been used, the 5-year spending limit would have totaled about $26 billion less. HHS established the largest portion of the Arizona spending limit, per person spending, using an outdated baseline of projections of the costs of operating the program without the demonstration.[46] The projections were based on the estimated costs of operating the program developed for the state's previous demonstration—initially approved in 1982—and adjusted forward to 2011. HHS's policy indicates that the spending limits for new demonstrations should be based on actual expenditures in the base year. Arizona's actual expenditures in 2011—the base year for the demonstration had HHS approved a spending limit based on its policy—were much lower than the projected costs used by HHS as the basis of the spending limit. HHS officials said that the agency was not able to estimate the cost of the Arizona Medicaid program without the demonstration using recent actual expenditure data, because the state's Medicaid program had operated under a demonstration since 1982. We found that HHS's rationale for relying on 30-year-old projections of what the Medicaid program would have cost without the demonstration was unsupported. Actual expenditure data were available and would more accurately reflect state spending under Medicaid than the old projections that were based on the state operating without a Medicaid program. We estimate that HHS's use of projected costs rather than actual expenditures for the base year increased the spending limit by about $22 billion.

---

[46]The limit on per person spending included specific limits for six populations included in the demonstration: those eligible on the basis of receiving Supplemental Security Income, persons with developmental disabilities, elderly and physically disabled persons, children and families, childless adults, and participants in the family planning program. In addition to the per person limit on spending, Arizona's spending limit also included $1.7 billion for the state to finance uncompensated care, about $77 million to expand coverage to children up to age 19 with family income up to 175 percent of the FPL not otherwise eligible for Medicaid, and unspecified amounts for other activities such as payments to Indian Health Service facilities.

HHS's approved spending limit for Arizona also used growth rates for certain populations that were higher than the benchmark growth rates suggested by agency policy.[47] The rates HHS used reflected national growth rates, which were higher than the state historical growth rates based on actual state historical expenditures. (See table 2.) Instead, HHS compared national growth rates to the projected state growth approved as part of the state's previous demonstration, developed 30 years earlier. Officials also told us that they did not consider comparing the national growth rates to the state's historical growth rates derived from actual state expenditures because it was unclear if these expenditures would have occurred absent the demonstration. However, without the demonstration, Arizona would not have a Medicaid program. In addition, the previously approved rate does not appear to be a valid substitute given the large difference between that rate and the growth rates indicated by actual historical expenditure data. We estimate that HHS's use of the previously projected growth rates rather than actual state expenditures to derive the benchmark growth rate increased the approved 5-year spending limit by about $4.2 billion.

Table 2: Comparison of Growth Rates Approved by the Department of Health and Human Services (HHS) for the Arizona Medicaid Demonstration and Benchmark Growth Rates

Percent

Medicaid beneficiary category	HHS-approved growth rate[a]	Benchmark growth rate
Persons receiving Supplemental Security Income	6.0%	4.4%
Persons with developmental disabilities	6.0	0.3
Elderly and physically disabled persons	5.2	2.6
Children and families	5.2	2.5

Source: GAO analysis of HHS data.

[a]Annual growth rates approved by HHS in October 2011 for the 5-year term of the demonstration (October 2011–September 2016).

---

[47]The exceptions were the per person spending limits for childless adults and for the family planning extension program. For childless adults, HHS approved a per person spending limit equal to the state's projection of per person costs in the first year of the demonstration and did not allow per person costs to grow for the population. For the family planning demonstration, HHS used the national growth rate, which was lower than the state historical growth rate.

Indiana

For the Indiana demonstration, HHS approved a spending limit that was based on a projected growth rate that exceeded the benchmark growth rate without clear support for doing so. Had HHS used the benchmark growth rate, the demonstration's 5-year spending limit would have been an estimated $416 million lower. While HHS developed growth rates based on only 3 of the 5 years of historical data, HHS documented that the most recent 2 years of data reflected large decreases in spending from the state's increased use of managed care and that these changes in spending were a onetime effect that likely would not continue. We determined that HHS had adequately explained and documented its reason for making this adjustment. However, we found that HHS did not have adequate support for approving a 4.4 percent growth rate for all four populations included in the demonstration, when the historical data provided by the state showed benchmark growth rates that were lower than 4.4 percent for three of those populations.[48] (See table 3.) HHS officials stated that a policy decision was made to use the average state historical growth rates because it was believed that it was more likely to reflect cost trends in the future. Officials added that one of the individual populations had a zero growth rate historically and it was decided that as a result of regular health care inflation, costs would grow. Approving an average growth rate does not appear to be a valid substitute for the state historical growth rates for each population given the significant difference for the adult caretaker populations, and the fact that health care inflation was present during prior years and would have also affected population-specific growth rates. Had HHS used benchmark growth rates for each population, the spending limit would have been about $416 million lower than the approved spending limit.

---

[48] The four populations include children, pregnant women, children's caretakers who have historically been eligible for Medicaid, and children's caretakers newly eligble for Medicaid under the demonstration.

Table 3: Comparison of Growth Rates Approved by the Department of Health and Human Services (HHS) for the Indiana Medicaid Demonstration and Benchmark Growth Rates

Percent

Medicaid beneficiary category	HHS-approved growth rate[a]	Benchmark growth rate
Children	4.4%	4.9%
Pregnant women	4.4	4.1
Historically eligible adult caretakers	4.4	0.0
Newly eligible adult caretakers	4.4	0.0

Source: GAO analysis of HHS data.

[a]Annual growth rates approved by HHS in December 2007 for the 5-year term of the demonstration. (January 2008–December 2012).

Rhode Island

HHS approved an aggregate spending limit of about $12.1 billion for the Rhode Island demonstration based on a growth rate that exceeded the benchmark growth rate without clearly supporting the use of a higher growth rate. Had HHS used the benchmark growth rate, we estimate that the spending limit would have been about $772 million lower than the approved limit. According to HHS officials, the spending limit was developed using the 2006 base year average national growth rate of 7.8 percent; however, the state's historical growth rate in the 5 years prior to applying for the demonstration was 7.0 percent. HHS officials told us that though the state provided data for 2007 to be used as the base year, HHS instead chose 2006 as the base year, because negative trends in the 2007 data were not representative, did not appear reliable, and contained what they called outliers. So while HHS based the Rhode Island spending limit on the lower of the two growth rates for 2006, the agency could not provide clear support for using that base year. (See table 4.)

Table 4: National and State-Historical Growth Rates that the Department of Health and Human Services (HHS) Compared in Selecting a Base Year and Approving the Rhode Island Medicaid Demonstration

Growth rates using 2006 as base year		Growth rates using 2007 as base year	
HHS-approved growth rate[a]	State historical growth rate	National growth rate	State-historical growth rate
7.8%	7.9%	8.0%	7.0%

Source: GAO analysis of HHS data.

[a]The HHS-approved growth rate in Rhode Island was the national growth rate (January 2009–December 2013).

Texas

In Texas, the HHS-approved spending limit included two types of hypothetical costs in the state's base year expenditures. These costs represented higher payment amounts the state could have paid to providers, but did not actually pay. We estimated that, had the state only included actual expenditures as indicated by HHS's policy, the spending limit would have totaled about $4.6 billion less. HHS's decision sets a precedent that a state can increase a demonstration spending limit on the basis that it could have hypothetically paid Medicaid providers more than it actually chose to pay them, without a clear basis for doing so.

First, Texas's spending limit was based, in part, on hypothetical costs as opposed to actual incurred expenditures with respect to UPL payments that could be made for inpatient hospital services but were not actually made. Prior to applying for this demonstration, about 1.3 million of the state's Medicaid population received inpatient hospital services under managed care, and the state did not make UPL payments for these services.[49] In its spending limit estimate, however, Texas included costs for UPL payments and fee-for-service payments for beneficiaries previously receiving inpatient hospital services under a managed care delivery model. In its proposal, the state said it would take certain actions in response to directives from its state legislature. Specifically, the state said that if the demonstration was not approved by HHS it would carve out inpatient hospital services previously provided under managed care and pay for these services on a fee-for-service basis and also make UPL payments for these services. These actions would increase costs because fee-for-service payments and UPL payments to hospitals would greatly exceed capitation payments made to managed care plans. HHS officials stated that, given a directive of the Texas legislature, they believed the state would do so, and they allowed the estimated increased costs of such an arrangement to be factored into the spending limit even though Texas had not changed its payment model. As a result, $3.8 billion of the demonstration spending limit was based on what Texas estimated it could pay providers in the future but had not been paying prior to the demonstration.

Second, Texas proposed including additional hypothetical costs in the base year expenditures by using the maximum amount of UPL payments

---

[49]As referenced above, states are generally prohibited from making supplemental payments for services delivered under a managed care payment and delivery model.

the state could have paid rather than the actual amount of payments the state did make. In its proposal, the state documented that during each of the 4 years leading up to and including the base year, the state's actual hospital inpatient UPL payments were less than the maximum amount the state could have paid.[50] HHS officials noted that because the actual payments were accounting for an increasing percentage of the maximum UPL payments the state could have made, they allowed the state to use this larger amount. As a result of HHS's decision, about $796 million of the demonstration spending limit was based on a hypothetical expenditure that did not represent actual expenditures of the state under its program.[51]

HHS Approved Spending Limits for Three Demonstrations Based on Actual DSH Expenditures and Followed Statutory Criteria in Approving Spending Limits for Three Other Demonstrations

HHS approved spending limits for three demonstrations that redirected federal DSH funds, which were consistent with its policy. For the District of Columbia, Missouri, and Wisconsin demonstrations, HHS limited federal spending to the lower of the states' DSH allotment or actual DSH expenditures in the year prior to the demonstrations.[52] This approach helps provide assurances that the federal government will spend no more under the demonstrations than what it would have spent without them. For the District of Columbia and Missouri, HHS limited federal spending to a specific dollar amount, which represented a portion of the states' DSH expenditures in the year prior to the demonstrations' approvals.[53] The

---

[50]As referenced above, the federal share of UPL payments are limited to a reasonable estimate of what Medicare would pay for a similar service.

[51]Although reviewing the accuracy of the state's calculation of the maximum UPL was not within the scope of our review, we have previously reported concerns with the different methods and data used by states to estimate the amount of UPL payments allowed. See GAO, *Medicaid: Improved Federal Oversight of State Financing Schemes Is Needed*, GAO-04-228 (Washington, D.C: Feb. 13, 2004). Further, UPL supplemental payment calculations are not subject to annual independent audits that verify that states have accurately calculated the maximum allowable UPL payments using reliable data, which is required for DSH payments. See GAO, *Medicaid: More Transparency of and Accountability for Supplemental Payments Are Needed*, GAO-13-48 (Washington, D.C.: Nov. 26, 2013). HHS officials said they did not review the state UPL calculation in reviewing and approving the state spending limits, and used the maximum payment amounts submitted by the state.

[52]Use of DSH allotments to set demonstration spending limits does not require the use of growth rates to project future costs.

[53]The remaining funds under the District of Columbia's and Missouri's allotments are available for the states to make DSH payments to hospitals.

Wisconsin spending limit was set at the total DSH allotment, which also represented the amount of expenditures in the year prior to the demonstration's approval. The approved spending limit for the entire length of the demonstration was about $145 million for the District of Columbia, $105 million for Missouri, and $797 million for Wisconsin.

The Idaho, Michigan, and New Mexico demonstrations were a unique type of section 1115 demonstration governed by requirements not applicable to other types of Medicaid section 1115 demonstrations. For these three states, HHS set spending limits using a process provided for under CHIPRA. These states applied and received approval for new section 1115 demonstrations, through which they continued to cover childless adults using Medicaid funds instead of CHIP funds. CHIPRA also defined the budget neutrality process for such demonstrations by identifying the base year and growth rates for demonstration spending limits.[54] For each of the three demonstrations, HHS followed the budget neutrality procedures outlined in CHIPRA in setting the spending limit on an annual basis. The initial annual spending limits were based on expenditure projections of about $80,000 for Idaho, about $137 million for Michigan, and about $177 million for New Mexico. For the first demonstration year, spending limits were slightly less because the demonstrations operated less than a full year.

HHS's Policy Does Not Reflect Current Processes or Provide Assurances That Data Used for Developing Spending Limits Are Reliable

HHS's policy for setting spending limits for proposed demonstrations is inconsistent with its actual practices. To this extent, HHS's internal controls are insufficient. According to *Standards for Internal Control in the Federal Government*, government processes, including management directives and administrative policies, should be clearly documented.[55] In discussing documentation for HHS's policy, published in 2001, officials indicated that it reflected HHS's most current processes and policy on

---

[54]CHIPRA required that HHS limit spending for fiscal year 2010 to the amount spent by the state for that population in fiscal year 2009 increased by the percentage increase (if any) between 2009 and 2010 in the projected nominal per capita amount of the National Health Expenditures. The act further required HHS to increase annual spending limits for the remaining years based on the percentage increase, if any, in the projected nominal per capita amount of the National Health Expenditures as published for each calendar year.

[55]GAO, *Standards for Internal Control in the Federal Government*, GAO/AIMD-00-21.3.1 (Washington, D.C.: November 1999).

budget neutrality, but acknowledged that some aspects of the policy, as written, were no longer applicable to current processes. For example, HHS officials told us that the methods described for determining spending limits of demonstration extensions were no longer applied. In addition, while the policy requires that states submit 5 years of historical data in developing spending limits—and HHS officials told us that this is their preference—the agency's current processes allow states to use data based on the state's estimate of spending or enrollment. For example, if the 2 most recent years of expenditure data are not available because of delays in Medicaid claims processing, estimates for these years can be used. Officials indicated that if estimates are used instead of actual data, the state must explain any adjustments. But HHS officials did not have documentation for the current process or policy on when estimates are allowed, or the type of documentation of adjustments that is required. In addition, the HHS's policy does not require documentation or describe how the data used to set spending limits are reviewed to ensure reliability and accuracy. According to officials, the data used for projecting spending comes from each state's Medicaid data system, and HHS generally does not test the accuracy of the data. However, officials noted that the state systems may have their own quality and reliability checks.

In October 2012, HHS introduced an optional waiver application template that included a standard budget neutrality form that states could use to submit 1115 demonstration applications.[56] The template provides a standard format for states to submit commonly used data elements—such as historical expenditure and enrollment data, and the projected growth rates and per capita costs based on the state historical enrollment and costs—and a description of the sources and methods for obtaining state historical data. The budget neutrality form allows states to submit actual or estimated data. HHS officials told us that the new template does not establish any new budget neutrality policy, but instead was intended to make the application template more user-friendly than the prior template that was developed in conjunction with the agency's policy published in 2001. The new budget neutrality form reiterates HHS's 2001 policy that states that spending limits should be based on the lower of the state-specific historical growth rate or estimated nationwide growth rate. The form does not provide additional guidance, for example, on the process and criteria for when estimated state historical data rather than actual

---

[56]This template was not in effect for the demonstrations we reviewed.

state historical expenditure data are used in setting spending limits, or when deviations from the benchmark policy are allowed and how they should be documented and supported.

Conclusions

The fiscal challenges facing the federal government require prudent stewardship of federal Medicaid resources. While section 1115 Medicaid demonstrations serve as an important mechanism for states to implement projects that allow for innovation while promoting Medicaid objectives, HHS policy requires that they not expose the federal government to additional financial liability. The Secretary of Health and Human Services has an important responsibility for ensuring that comprehensive demonstrations will not increase federal costs above what would be incurred without these demonstrations. HHS's long-standing budget neutrality policy for these demonstrations, on its face, recognizes that states should not be given access to additional federal funding at the same time they are provided with greater program flexibility. However, neither the policy, nor HHS's implementation of it, ensures the prudent stewardship of federal Medicaid spending.

After examining HHS's approach for approving spending limits of recently approved demonstrations, we have three main concerns regarding the budget neutrality policy and process. First, HHS's policy is not reflected in its actual practices and, contrary to sound management practices, is not adequately documented. Second, the policy and processes lack transparency regarding criteria and the supporting evidence required to justify deviations from historical spending and established benchmark growth rates. We recognize that forecasting spending during changing economic times is challenging and a state's circumstances may warrant such deviations. Nonetheless, we believe that approved spending limits that are based on baselines and growth rate expectations that greatly deviate from HHS's current benchmarks should be well-supported and documented. HHS's policy is currently silent as to when deviations are allowed and does not require that reliable evidence be provided to justify deviations. Transparency around the basis for spending limit decisions is important not only for assurances of the ongoing fiscal integrity and sustainability of the program, but also for assurances of consistency of approvals among states. Third, the policy as implemented allows methods for establishing spending limits that we believe are inappropriate for such purposes, such as allowing states to include hypothetical costs in the baseline for spending limits. The second and third concerns parallel those we have raised in earlier reports. In 2008, because HHS disagreed that changes to the budget neutrality policy and review process were needed, we suggested that Congress consider requiring increased attention to fiscal responsibility in the approval of section 1115 Medicaid demonstrations and require the Secretary of Health and Human Services to improve the demonstration review process by, for example, clarifying the criteria for approving spending limits and documenting and making public the basis for such approvals. Thus far Congress has not acted on this suggestion. On the basis of the findings in this report, we believe the Secretary needs to take additional actions to ensure that HHS's budget neutrality policy reflects current practices and that the spending limits for the Texas and Arizona demonstrations are appropriate, well supported, and based on clear criteria.

Recommendations for Executive Action

To improve the transparency of the process for reviewing and approving spending limits for comprehensive section 1115 demonstrations, we recommend that the Secretary of Health and Human Services take the following two actions:

1. update the agency's written budget neutrality policy to reflect actual criteria and processes used to develop and approve demonstration spending limits, and ensure the policy is readily available to state Medicaid directors and others; and

2. reconsider adjustments and costs used in setting the spending limits for the Arizona and Texas demonstrations, and make appropriate adjustments to spending limits for the remaining years of each demonstration.

Agency Comments and Our Evaluation

We provided a draft of this report to HHS for comment. In its written comments, HHS acknowledged that it has not always communicated its budget neutrality policy broadly or clearly, but stated it has applied its policy consistently. The Department suggested that recent steps to increase transparency—such as publishing a new section 1115 application template and implementing a federal public input process—reflect updated policy on how HHS sets spending limits and ensures demonstrations are budget neutral. While the application template may contain guidance on some of the data elements commonly used to demonstrate budget neutrality, we do not believe that it addresses how HHS reviews the applications or the criteria used for setting spending limits. We have revised our report to clarify how this template falls short of clarifying HHS's budget neutrality policy. HHS did not otherwise identify any written policy it has issued since 2001 either during the course of our review or in its comments.

HHS did not concur with our recommendation that its budget neutrality policy should be updated to reflect the actual criteria and processes used to develop and approve demonstration spending limits, and ensure that the policy is readily available. HHS stated that our findings that four states' spending limits would have been lower had the agency followed its policy were flawed. HHS said that we used only a subset of the best available data that the Department used to assess budget neutrality and that we relied on an outdated policy issued in 2001. We disagree with these assertions. It is important to note that, to do our analysis, we relied on extensive documentation and information that HHS officials specifically provided us as the basis for the selected states' budget neutrality determinations. For example, we obtained the spreadsheets with the data and calculations that HHS used to determine each state's demonstration spending limits. We reconciled these spreadsheets with the spending limits and documentation in each state's demonstration approval and had numerous discussions with HHS officials to confirm our understanding of the data and the basis for the final spending limits. At no time did officials tell us that they had provided us only with a subset of the data used to assess budget neutrality or cite additional information or data that we had not considered. HHS's assertion that we relied on an outdated budget neutrality policy that did not reflect the Department's current policy also conflicts with information provided to us during the course of this review. On multiple occasions, we discussed with officials the policy used to establish demonstration spending limits, including the applicability of the 2001 written policy. HHS officials told us—both verbally and in writing—that the 2001 written policy generally reflected the Department's current policy toward budget neutrality. They told us that this document was the most recent document capturing the budget neutrality policy. However, as we described in the draft report, HHS officials told us that some parts of the 2001 written policy were outdated. The Department did not have any plans to update the 2001 policy.

HHS did not concur with our recommendation that it should make adjustments to the spending limits for the remaining years of the Arizona and Texas demonstrations. In its comments, HHS said that the adjustments and costs it used were justified. However, HHS did not provide any new information or support beyond what was considered and discussed in the draft report. For example, HHS did not respond to our concerns that Texas' spending limit included $3.8 billion in costs that the state could hypothetically pay providers in the future but did not actually pay them prior to the demonstration. We continue to believe HHS' decisions were not clear or well supported. HHS also stated that it had significantly strengthened the accountability in Texas by requiring HHS approval before federal matching funds can be drawn down for state expenditures made under the demonstration, and by instituting robust reporting requirements. We believe that improved oversight of actual spending occurring under the demonstrations does not lessen the need for establishing sound spending limits.

HHS's comments are reproduced in appendix III. HHS also provided technical comments, which we incorporated as appropriate.

As agreed with your office, unless you publicly announce the contents of this report earlier, we plan no further distribution until 30 days from the report date. At that time, we will send copies of this report to the Secretary of Health and Human Services. In addition, the report is available at no charge on the GAO website at http://www.gao.gov.

If you or your staff have any questions about this report, please contact me at (202) 512-7114 or iritanik@gao.gov. Contact points for our Offices of Congressional Relations and Public Affairs may be found on the last page of this report. Major contributors to this report are listed in appendix IV.

Sincerely yours,

Katherine M. Iritani
Director, Health Care

Appendix I: Summary of Submitted and Reviewed Applications for Comprehensive Section 1115 Medicaid Demonstrations

From January 2007 through May 2012, the Department of Health and Human Services (HHS) received 62 comprehensive section 1115 Medicaid demonstration applications from 38 states, 3 of which were subsequently withdrawn by the states. HHS approved 45 of the remaining applications, disapproved 1, and another 13 were still pending completion of review as of May 31, 2012.[1] About two-thirds, or 31, of the 45 approved applications were for extensions of existing demonstrations, while 8 of the 13 still under review were for new demonstrations. For the 46 reviews that HHS completed, reviews took from 47 days to almost 4 years, and averaged 323 days from the date of application to the date of the review decision.[2] About 72 percent of the reviews took a year or less to complete. (See table 5.)

---

[1] We excluded from our review demonstrations that were not comprehensive, that is, they were limited to one category of services. We also excluded demonstrations that extended coverage to new populations in response to Medicaid expansion, as provided for under the Patient Protection and Affordable Care Act (PPACA).

[2] The review times we report are based on the number of calendar days between the date when HHS received an official application and the date HHS made its final decision on whether to approve or not approve the application. Review times do not include any preliminary discussions and reviews of concept papers.

Appendix I: Summary of Submitted and
Reviewed Applications for Comprehensive
Section 1115 Medicaid Demonstrations

Table 5: Status of Comprehensive Section 1115 Medicaid Demonstration Applications, by State, Submitted to the Department of Health and Human Services (HHS) from January 2007 through May 2012

State	Demonstration name	Application date	Decision date	Days between application and decision
AR	Arkansas Safety Net Benefit Program	9/29/10	12/29/11	456
AR	Arkansas ARKidsB	12/18/07	12/23/10	1,101
AR	Arkansas TEFRA-like	6/01/10	12/14/10	196
AZ	Arizona Health Care Cost Containment System[a]	3/31/11	10/21/11	204
CA	California Bridge to Reform	6/03/10	11/02/10	152
CO	Colorado Adults without Dependent Children	12/02/11	3/30/12	119
CO	Colorado Adult Prenatal Coverage and Premium Assistance in CHP+	5/27/09	Pending	Pending
DC	District of Columbia Childless Adults[a]	7/23/10	10/28/10	97
DE	Delaware Diamond State Health Plan	7/01/09	1/31/11	579
FL	Florida Medicaid Reform	6/30/10	12/15/11	533
FL	Florida MEDS-AD	12/30/09	12/14/10	349
HI	Hawaii QUEST Expanded	2/17/07	2/07/08	355
IA	Iowa Care	10/09/09	09/01/10	327
ID	Idaho Children's Access Card	8/04/09	9/30/10	422
ID	Idaho Non-pregnant Childless Adults (Idaho Adult Access Card Demonstration)[a]	9/09/09	12/23/09	105
IL	Illinois New Demo Program	1/30/12	Pending	Pending
IN	Healthy Indiana Plan[a]	7/03/07	12/14/07	164
IN	Healthy Indiana Plan	12/28/11	Pending	Pending
KS	Kansas Kan Care[b]	Withdrawn	Withdrawn	Withdrawn
KY	Kentucky Health Care Partnership	10/29/10	11/17/11	384
LA	Louisiana Greater New Orleans Community Health Connection	8/06/10	9/22/10	47
MA	MassHealth	6/30/10	12/20/11	538
MD	Maryland Health Choice	7/01/10	6/27/11	361
ME	Maine Childless Adults	9/30/09	9/27/10	362
MI	Michigan Medicaid Nonpregnant Childless Adults Waiver (Adults Benefit Waiver)[a]	9/29/09	12/22/09	84
MN	Minnesota Long Term Care Realignment	2/13/12	Pending	Pending
MN	Minnesota Prepaid Medical Assistance Project Plus	6/29/10	6/30/11	366
MO	Missouri Gateway to Better Health[a]	2/16/10	7/28/10	162
MS	Healthier Mississippi	9/29/08	10/28/10	759
MT	Montana Basic Medicaid for Able Bodied Adults	1/25/08	11/24/10	1,034
MT	Montana Medicaid Pharmacy Part D	1/28/11	6/17/11	140
NJ	New Jersey Comprehensive Waiver	9/9/11	Pending	Pending

Appendix I: Summary of Submitted and
Reviewed Applications for Comprehensive
Section 1115 Medicaid Demonstrations

State	Demonstration name	Application date	Decision date	Days between application and decision
NJ	New Jersey Childless Adults	2/24/11	4/14/11	49
NJ	New Jersey Family Coverage Under SCHIP	9/30/08	8/13/12	1,413
NM	New Mexico State Coverage Insurance–Title XIX Component[a]	9/28/09	12/30/09	93
NM	New Mexico State Coverage Insurance–Title XXI Component	9/24/10	2/18/11	147
NM	New Mexico State Coverage Insurance–Title XXI Component	5/1/12	Pending	Pending
NM	New Mexico Title XXI SCHIP	12/29/09	12/16/10	352
NM	New Mexico Centennial Care-New 1115[b]	Withdrawn	Withdrawn	Withdrawn
NV	Nevada Comprehensive Care Waiver	4/24/12	Pending	Pending
NY	New York State's People First Waiver	11/04/11	Pending	Pending
NY	New York Federal-State Health Reform Partnership	9/30/10	3/31/11	182
NY	New York Partnership Plan	3/31/09	7/29/11	850
OH	Ohio Transformation	4/26/12	Pending	Pending
OK	Oklahoma SoonerCare	6/30/09	12/30/09	183
OK	Oklahoma SoonerCare	12/30/11	Pending	Pending
OR	Oregon Health Plan	10/22/09	3/17/10	146
OR	Oregon Health Plan	2/29/12	Pending	Pending
RI	Rhode Island Global Consumer Choice Compact[a]	8/08/08	1/16/09	161
TN	TennCare II	6/15/09	12/15/09	183
TX	Texas Healthcare Transformation and Quality Improvement Program[a]	7/15/11	12/12/11	150
TX	Texas Health Care Reform Section 1115 Demonstration[c]	Withdrawn	Withdrawn	Withdrawn
UT	Utah Medicaid Payment and Service Delivery Reform	6/30/11	Pending	Pending
UT	Utah Primary Care Network	3/01/10	6/23/10	114
VA	Virginia FAMIS MOMS and FAMIS Select	10/15/09	6/29/10	257
VT	Vermont Global Commitment to Health	9/29/09	12/29/10	456
VT	Vermont Choices for Care	6/17/10	9/21/10	96
WA	Washington Transitional Bridge Demonstration	7/07/10	1/03/11	180
WI	Wisconsin BadgerCare Plus for Childless Adults[a]	7/01/08	12/31/08	183
WI	Wisconsin BadgerCare	9/28/10	12/30/10	93
WI	Wisconsin Senior Care	2/9/09	8/17/09	189
WI	Wisconsin Medicaid 2014	11/10/11	Pending	Pending

Source: GAO analysis of Centers for Medicare & Medicaid Services (CMS) data.

Notes: All of the demonstrations for which the review process was completed were approved with the exception of the Montana Medicaid Pharmacy Part D demonstration. Applications marked as pending had not been fully reviewed by HHS as of May 31, 2012.

[a]This is 1 of the 10 new approved comprehensive demonstrations that we reviewed.

[b]Application was withdrawn and subsequently resubmitted after May 31, 2012, which exceeded the time frame covered by this report.

[c]State withdrew application after HHS raised concerns about the state's proposal.

**Appendix I: Summary of Submitted and
Reviewed Applications for Comprehensive
Section 1115 Medicaid Demonstrations**

Officials with HHS stated that the nature of demonstration reviews is unpredictable because of the different factors outside HHS's control, which can influence the review. Further, HHS generally does not have a set time frame within which applications must be reviewed.[3] There are a number of factors that may have affected the review times for the demonstrations we reviewed.[4] For example, prior to applying for a new demonstration, states may submit a concept paper to HHS to receive technical assistance, advice, and other guidance. There may then be extended dialogue between a state and HHS about the plans included in a concept paper. The process can provide states with an initial indication of the acceptability of their proposal and thereby facilitate the application process. According to the officials, in cases where states have submitted such papers, HHS reviews may be shorter. In addition, the purpose, scale, and complexity of demonstration applications vary, and will result in the need for more or less discussion between the state and HHS. Similarly, the completeness of the application can affect review times. Applications may have lacked important details, such as data on how the program will be implemented, its effect on relevant beneficiary populations, or how budget neutrality is achieved. In these cases HHS may request extensive clarification, which adds to the review time because of the time states need to respond. Also, HHS officials said that state legislative activity can alter the proposal during development, or midcourse, which would extend HHS review times.

---

[3] Section 1115 of the Social Security Act does impose time frames for the review of certain extensions. Specifically, states are required to submit applications for extensions at least 120 days prior to the expiration date of the demonstration. HHS is required to either approve or disapprove these extensions within 120 days after submission of the applications. 42 U.S.C. § 1315(f). This process, however, only applies to extensions that do not seek to change the terms and conditions of the original demonstrations. HHS officials informed us that all of the extensions referenced in table 5 contained significant changes to the terms and conditions and therefore were treated as new applications, which do not have any applicable time frames for review.

[4] Review times may be affected in the future by recent HHS regulations. PPACA, enacted in 2010, required the Secretary of Health and Human Services to issue regulations for section 1115 applications that address certain topics including a state and federal public notice and comment process, submission of reports on implementation by states, and periodic evaluation by HHS. In response, on February 27, 2012, HHS published final regulations establishing these requirements, some of which may affect HHS review times. For example, after receipt of a completed application, HHS must provide for a 30-day public comment period and has to wait at least 45 days before making a final decision. These requirements apply to applications submitted on or after April 27, 2012, and therefore do not apply to the applications we are addressing in this report.

Appendix II: A Summary of Key Features of Recent Demonstrations

This appendix summarizes key information on 10 new comprehensive section 1115 demonstrations approved from January 2007 through May 2012. Key information presented includes: a summary of specific details about the purpose of the demonstration; the population covered; the term of each demonstration; the estimated number of people covered in the first and last year of the demonstration; and the approved spending limit over the term of each demonstration.[1] Because the scope and purpose of demonstrations vary by state, the amount and detail of the information provided for each demonstration also varies.

Arizona Health Care Cost Containment System

Demonstration Term: October 2011–September 2016

Estimated Number of People Covered: first year: 1,129,869; last year: 1,806,984

Approved Spending Limit: Over $74.4 billion

Arizona requested to terminate its previous section 1115 demonstration, operating since 1982, in order to eliminate coverage for one of its adult populations covered previously, and to implement an enrollment freeze on its childless adults, effective in July 2011. The population that was to be eliminated was covered through the Medical Expense Deduction program, which was for adults with income in excess of 100 percent of the federal poverty level (FPL) who have qualifying health care costs that reduce their income to or below 40 percent of the FPL. The enrollment freeze applied to adults without dependent children with family income up to and including 100 percent of the FPL. This new demonstration continued to provide coverage for the Medicaid population through managed care. In addition, the state was approved to establish state a funding pool for making supplemental payments, totaling over $300 million per year, to providers that cover Medicaid and uncompensated care costs, and to make hospital payments for trauma and emergency services through a program that was originally a state-funded initiative. The demonstration also expanded coverage to certain children up to age 19 and women who lose Medicaid pregnancy

---

[1]We reported the estimated number of people covered and the approved spending limit when it was clearly stated in the approval documents. When it was not clearly stated, we estimated these figures using information from the approval documents.

Appendix II: A Summary of Key Features of Recent Demonstrations

coverage.[2] The state increased personal financial responsibility through cost sharing by implementing the use of penalties for certain enrollees that miss scheduled physician appointments, and encouraging appropriate utilization of emergency room care by imposing cost sharing for improper use of the emergency room.[3] The state also imposed higher cost sharing for brand name drugs when a generic is available.[4]

District of Columbia Childless Adults

Demonstration Term: November 2010–December 2013

Estimated Number of People Covered: first year: 4,815; last year: 11,121

Approved Spending Limit: $145 million

The District of Columbia was approved to redirect Disproportionate Share Hospital (DSH) funds in order to provide full Medicaid benefits to adults ages 21 through 64 with incomes between 133 percent and 200 percent of the FPL. Benefits under the demonstration were provided through a mandatory managed care delivery system. Most anticipated enrollees were covered previously through a local program that provided more limited benefits.

---

[2]Coverage is for children up to age 19 with family income up to 175 percent of the FPL not otherwise eligible for Medicaid and pregnancy coverage is extended for up to 24 months after birth.

[3]Nonemergency use of the emergency room can cost enrollees $30.

[4]The cost for a brand-name drug is $10 compared to $4 for a generic drug.

Appendix II: A Summary of Key Features of
Recent Demonstrations

Idaho Nonpregnant Childless Adults (Idaho Adult Access Card Demonstration)

Demonstration Term: January 2010–September 2014

Estimated Number of People Covered: first year: 350; last year: 350

Approved Spending Limit:[5] $596,476

Idaho was approved under a new demonstration to continue to provide premium subsidies to nonpregnant childless adults age 18 and above with incomes at or below 185 percent of the FPL.[6] The demonstration allows a premium subsidy up to $100 per month per enrolled adult—a qualifying employee or the spouse of the employee—toward the individual's share of the employer-sponsored health insurance premium. Participating employers are required to make a 50 percent contribution toward the cost of the health benefit plan.

Healthy Indiana Plan

Demonstration Term: January 2008–December 2012

Estimated Number of People Covered: first year: 669,894; last year: 848,919

Approved Spending Limit: $10.6 billion

Indiana received approval to operate two distinct health insurance programs. This demonstration preserved the program previously in place for Medicaid-eligible individuals and expanded coverage to uninsured adults; both programs were run through a managed care delivery system. The first program, called the Hoosier Healthwise Program, continued coverage for current Medicaid-eligible individuals. The second program, called Healthy Indiana Plan (HIP), expanded coverage for uninsured adults, not currently eligible for Medicaid. The expansion was partially funded using redirected DSH funding. The HIP provided a high-deductible health plan and an account similar to a health savings account for uninsured adults including low-income custodial parents and caretaker

---

[5]We estimated the total federal and state costs using the 2012 federal medical assistance percentage (FMAP).

[6]Idaho was required by federal law to discontinue using the State Children's Health Insurance Program (CHIP) funds to cover childless adults, but was allowed to continue services for this population with Medicaid funds under a new section 1115 demonstration.

Appendix II: A Summary of Key Features of
Recent Demonstrations

relatives of Medicaid and State Children's Health Insurance Program (CHIP) children, and uninsured noncustodial parents and childless adults ages 19 through 64 with incomes between 22 and 200 percent of the FPL.

Participation in HIP is voluntary, but all enrollees are required to receive medical care through the high-deductible health plans. HIP enrollees are required to help fund the $1,100 deductible by contributing to a savings account.[7] These accounts are used by enrollees to pay for the cost of health care services until the deductible is reached; however, preventive services up to a maximum amount are exempt from this requirement. The benefits available under HIP are limited to $300,000 annually, and $1 million over a lifetime. The demonstration also included cost sharing depending on income.

Michigan Childless Adults Waiver

Demonstration Term: January 2010–September 2014

Estimated Number of People Covered: first year: 74,379; last year: 90,665

Approved Spending Limit:[8] $1 billion

Michigan was approved under a new demonstration to continue providing a limited ambulatory benefit package through a managed care delivery system to low-income nonpregnant childless adults ages 19 through 64 years with incomes at or below 35 percent of the FPL.[9] The benefit package included outpatient hospital services, physician services, diagnostic services, pharmacy, mental health and substance abuse services. Enrollees may be required to receive prior authorization before accessing certain ambulatory services.

---

[7]The contribution amounts range from 2 to 5 percent of income based on household income.

[8]We estimated the total federal and state costs using the 2012 federal medical assistance percentage (FMAP).

[9]Michigan was required by federal law to discontinue using CHIP funds to cover childless adults, but was allowed to continue services for this population with Medicaid funds under a new section 1115 demonstration.

Appendix II: A Summary of Key Features of Recent Demonstrations

Missouri Gateway to Better Health

Demonstration Term: July 2010–December 2013

Estimated Number of People Covered:[10] not available

Approved Spending Limit: $105 million

Missouri was approved to redirect its DSH funding to pay for four main activities in the St. Louis area: (1) health clinics that will provide services to the uninsured; (2) a health commission to manage activities related to the demonstration; and (3) a program to educate and encourage patients to use primary care rather than the emergency room. Lastly, the state was approved to expand coverage through a pilot that provides limited primary care benefits and a voucher system to provide acute hospital services to a population in the St. Louis area.

New Mexico State Coverage Insurance—Title XIX Component

Demonstration Term: January 2010–September 2014

Estimated Number of People Covered:[11] 29,770

Approved Spending Limit: $1.3 billion

New Mexico was approved under a new demonstration to continue to provide coverage for nonpregnant childless adults.[12] The eligible population is nonpregnant childless adults ages 19 to 64 years with incomes up to and including 200 percent of the FPL who are not eligible for Medicaid. Enrollees receive a comprehensive benefit package through a managed care delivery system in which premiums and copayments are required. These premiums include up to $35 for higher-income childless adults. The demonstration was designed to provide health care coverage

---

[10]Information to estimate the number of people covered was not provided in the approval documentation.

[11]The state estimated that the demonstration would continue coverage for about 29,000 childless adults. However, information to estimate the number of people covered for the first and last year of the demonstration was not provided.

[12]New Mexico was required by federal law to discontinue using CHIP funds to cover childless adults, but was allowed to continue services for this population with Medicaid funds under a new section 1115 demonstration.

Appendix II: A Summary of Key Features of Recent Demonstrations

to uninsured individuals who are unemployed, self-employed, or employed by an employer with 50 or fewer employees.

Rhode Island Global Consumer Choice Compact

Demonstration Term: January 2009–December 2013

Estimated Number of People Covered: first year: 192,778; last year: 206,540

Approved Spending Limit: $12.1 billion

Rhode Island was approved to operate its entire Medicaid program under a demonstration and to continue to provide coverage to populations that were previously covered under several distinct waivers.[13] Rhode Island was allowed to redesign its Medicaid program to provide cost-effective services that will ensure beneficiaries receive the appropriate services in the least restrictive and most appropriate setting. For example, the state was allowed to form and pay for entities dedicated to reviewing the needs of enrollees eligible for long-term care. This organization helps enrollees decide how to manage their health care needs based on a distinction given to them as "highest need," "high need," or "preventive." This designation allows the state to determine which cost-effective long-term services an enrollee can receive. For example, those designated as highest-need individuals are approved to receive nursing home care while those designated as preventive are approved to receive certain home health services. The state was also approved to include other services under the demonstration, such as parenting and childbirth education classes, tobacco cessation services, and window replacement for lead-poisoned children.

---

[13] These populations were previously covered under the state plan, a different section 1115 demonstration, and other waivers including 1915(c) waivers.

Appendix II: A Summary of Key Features of Recent Demonstrations

Texas Healthcare Transformation and Quality Improvement Program

Demonstration Term: December 2011–September 2016

Estimated Number of People Covered: first year: 3,872,680; last year: 4,767,680

Approved Spending Limit: $142 Billion

The Texas demonstration allowed the state to both expand the use of a managed care delivery system to existing covered populations and to preserve supplemental payments through the establishment of funding pools. The state was allowed to claim approximately $29 billion over the 5-year term of the demonstration on these pool payments. One pool was used to reimburse providers for uncompensated care costs, and the other was used to provide incentive payments to participating hospitals that implement and operate delivery system reforms.[14] The state also was approved to cover children's primary and preventive Medicaid dental services through a capitated statewide dental services program.

Wisconsin BadgerCare Plus for Childless Adults

Demonstration Term: January 2009–December 2013

Estimated Number of People Covered: first year: 25,129; last year: 40,800

Approved Spending Limit: $797 million

Wisconsin obtained approval to redirect its DSH funding to expand coverage to childless adults, who are defined as individuals between the ages of 19 and 64 years with income that does not exceed 200 percent of the FPL. The program included a variety of features: a requirement for

---

[14]The incentive payments were intended to help the state and health care providers prepare for the expected increase in population after the Medicaid expansion under the Patient Protection and Affordable Care Act (PPACA) is fully implemented in 2014. At the time Texas's demonstration was approved, PPACA required all states to expand Medicaid coverage to a broader category of low-income individuals beginning in January of 2014. However, subsequent to this approval, a ruling by the U.S. Supreme Court essentially made the expansion a choice for the states. See *National Federation of Independent Business, et al., vs. Sebelius, Sec. of Health and Human Services, et al.*, 132 S. Ct. 2566 567 (U.S. June 28, 2012). In July of 2012, the Governor of Texas sent a letter to HHS stating that the state did not intend to expand Medicaid. In addition, in June 2013, a state law was enacted that would prohibit the state Medicaid agency from expanding Medicaid coverage.

Appendix II: A Summary of Key Features of Recent Demonstrations

participants to complete a health needs assessment—used to match enrollees with health maintenance organizations and providers that meet the individual's specific health care needs; tiering of health plans based on quality of care indicators; and enhanced online and telephone application tools that allow childless adults to choose from a variety of health insurance options.

Appendix III: Comments from the Department of Health and Human Services

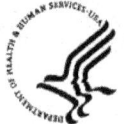

DEPARTMENT OF HEALTH & HUMAN SERVICES

OFFICE OF THE SECRETARY

Assistant Secretary for Legislation
Washington, DC 20201

MAY 3 1 2013

Katherine Iritani
Director, Health Care
U.S. Government Accountability Office
441 G Street NW
Washington, DC 20548

Dear Ms. Iritani

Attached are comments on the U.S. Government Accountability Office's (GAO) report entitled, entitle, "MEDICAID DEMONSTRATION WAIVERS: Approval Process Raises Cost Concerns and Lacks Transparency" (GAO-13-384).

The Department appreciates the opportunity to review this report prior to publication.

Sincerely,

Jim R. Esquea
Assistant Secretary for Legislation

Attachment

Appendix III: Comments from the Department of Health and Human Services

GENERAL COMMENTS OF THE DEPARTMENT OF HEALTH AND HUMAN SERVICES (HHS) ON THE GOVERNMENT ACCOUNTABILITY OFFICE'S (GAO) DRAFT REPORT ENTITLED, "MEDICAID DEMONSTRATION WAIVERS: APPROVAL PROCESS RAISES CONCERNS AND LACKS TRANSPARENCY" (GAO-13-384)

The Department appreciates the opportunity to review and comment on this draft report.

As GAO notes, budget neutrality as applied to section 1115 demonstrations is not required by law, but rather is a policy that HHS has applied over the years to ensure that federal expenditures under such demonstrations do not exceed what the federal government would have spent in the Medicaid program absent the demonstration. There are, as GAO points out, different ways that budget neutrality can be calculated. While we agree that budget neutrality policy has not always been conveyed as broadly and clearly as it could have been, the agency's policy has been consistently applied over the years.

Moreover, over the last period of time, HHS has taken new steps to make our approach to budget neutrality more transparent. On October 5, 2012, CMS released a section 1115 template for states to use in order to clarify the requirements and simplify the application process. This template includes instructions and an accompanying budget worksheet that provides guidance on some of the most commonly used data elements for demonstrating budget neutrality. Consistent with CMS' policy that budget neutrality calculations should be based on the best available data, states must provide an explanation of how the demonstration program will achieve budget neutrality and include data that supports the state's rationale. This guidance had not previously been communicated in this format and is part of the agency's broader effort to increase transparency in section 1115 demonstrations.

The section 1115 demonstration template is only one component of a broader set of recent initiatives that CMS has undertaken to improve transparency and the quality of care provided under demonstrations, while at the same time ensuring accountability for demonstration expenditures. For example, the Texas section 1115 demonstration reviewed by GAO includes detailed protocols and evaluation and monitoring criteria to guide the implementation of the demonstration and ensure accountability for the associated expenditures (for more information see http://medicaid.gov/Medicaid-CHIP-Program-Information/By-Topics/Waivers/1115/downloads/tx/tx-healthcare-transformation-ca.pdf).

In addition, CMS launched a new section on the Medicaid.gov website to receive public comments on demonstration applications and renewals and provide the public with all relevant demonstration documents, including budget neutrality agreements: (http://medicaid.gov/Medicaid-CHIP-Program-Information/By-Topics/Waivers/Waivers.html). Another example of CMS' focus on quality and accountability is the recently released series of tools and guidance on implementing managed care amendments to 1115 demonstrations that include long-term services and supports (see http://medicaid.gov/Medicaid-CHIP-Program-Information/By-Topics/Long-Term-Services-and-Support/Long-Term-Services-and-Support.html).

These changes and additional tools have assisted CMS in its consistent application of budget neutrality policy by adding to the transparency of the process and enhancing understanding between CMS and the states.

Appendix III: Comments from the Department of Health and Human Services

GENERAL COMMENTS OF THE DEPARTMENT OF HEALTH AND HUMAN SERVICES (HHS) ON THE GOVERNMENT ACCOUNTABILITY OFFICE'S (GAO) DRAFT REPORT ENTITLED, "MEDICAID DEMONSTRATION WAIVERS: APPROVAL PROCESS RAISES CONCERNS AND LACKS TRANSPARENCY" (GAO-13-384)

GAO Recommendation

HHS should update the agency's written budget neutrality policy to reflect the actual criteria and processes used to develop and approve demonstration spending limits and ensure the policy is readily available to state Medicaid directors and others.

HHS Response

HHS does not concur with GAO's assertion that HHS's budget neutrality policy and process do not assure that all recently approved demonstrations will be budget neutral.

GAO estimates that if HHS "had held the four demonstrations' spending to levels suggested by its policy" the 5-year spending limits should have been lower. This conclusion is flawed. First, in coming to its conclusion, GAO used only a subset of the data that CMS uses to assess budget neutrality and to determine the appropriate trend rate and estimates used in assessing budget neutrality.

Second, GAO relied on a very narrow reading of HHS's budget neutrality policy as a result of focusing on outdated written guidance provided in a letter to state Medicaid directors issued in 2001 for a different purpose (the letter related to a particular waiver approach known as the Health Insurance Flexibility and Accountability initiative). The 2001 letter was released to explain a specific policy established at the time and CMS no longer relies on this guidance in its review and approval of section 1115 demonstrations.

As noted previously, HHS policy is to use the best available data in determining the appropriate trend rate to estimate what expenditures would have been without a demonstration. Generally, that means using the lower of either the state's historical spending trend rate, or the President's budget trend rate, unless the state supplies compelling justification that another trend rate would be more appropriate. For example, in light of the recent economic downturn, in some cases CMS has determined that recent state trend rates are not an accurate indicator of what a state would have spent in future years in the absence of a waiver. During the downturn, many states took a variety of steps to reduce expenditures, for example, by cutting provider payment rates or reducing benefits. These actions were, in some instances, never intended to be permanent; and thus, we accounted for cyclical changes in spending by examining other relevant state data in establishing the "without waiver" baseline. As GAO notes "forecasting spending during changing economic times is challenging and a state's circumstances may warrant such deviations." As the report notes, it is also important to underscore that budget neutrality calculations set only the upper limits on the federal funds available to states under the demonstration; in order to claim federal matching funds, states must submit evidence of actual expenditures that are permissible under the terms of the demonstration.

Appendix III: Comments from the Department of Health and Human Services

GENERAL COMMENTS OF THE DEPARTMENT OF HEALTH AND HUMAN SERVICES (HHS) ON THE GOVERNMENT ACCOUNTABILITY OFFICE'S (GAO) DRAFT REPORT ENTITLED, "MEDICAID DEMONSTRATION WAIVERS: APPROVAL PROCESS RAISES CONCERNS AND LACKS TRANSPARENCY" (GAO-13-384)

GAO Recommendation

HHS should reconsider adjustments and costs used in setting the spending limits for the Arizona and Texas demonstrations and make appropriate adjustments to spending limits for the remaining years of each demonstration.

HHS Response

HHS does not concur with GAO's recommendation to reconsider the Arizona and Texas demonstration spending limits. As is explained in more detail below, CMS' calculation of these states' spending limits was consistent with longstanding policy and was based on the most reasonable and documented cost assumptions available regarding the interventions operationalized under the demonstration. In addition, for the reasons discussed below, HHS does not believe GAO's assumption that using different numbers for the budget neutrality calculations would have produced additional savings.

Arizona's section 1115 demonstration began in 1982, which coincided with the establishment of a Medicaid program in that state. Indeed, Arizona's Medicaid program is synonymous with the Arizona Health Care Cost Containment System demonstration. Because of the unique circumstances of the Arizona demonstration, CMS was not able to analyze expenditures during a pre-demonstration period to determine actual "without waiver" expenditures – there were no state Medicaid expenditures prior to 1982. In this situation, CMS determined that using the "without waiver" per member per month (PMPM) cost figures and corresponding trend rates approved under the previous demonstration was the best method for determining the "without waiver" PMPMs and trend rates for the new demonstration. HHS acknowledges GAO's recommendation that actual expenditures and trend rates could have been used, but they too would have raised issues because it is unclear whether these expenditures would have occurred absent the demonstration. CMS's approach to budget neutrality has been applied consistently – and transparently – for Arizona throughout the course of its demonstration.

The GAO report also questions CMS's decision to include potential costs in the budget neutrality baseline for the Texas Healthcare Transformation and Quality Improvement Program demonstration. CMS believes that the adjustments made to Texas' historical data are justified. The state Medicaid agency was required by state legislation to take necessary action to preserve supplemental payments to hospitals as it moved to greater use of managed care. The legislation provided that without demonstration authority to provide supplemental payments, the state would carve out inpatient hospital services from the existing STAR program benefits and pay fee-for-service for those benefits. Texas already had a model for accomplishing this, as the state had previously carved out inpatient hospital benefits from some of its existing STAR+ managed care programs to allow the state to continue to make supplemental payments. Since this was the most likely scenario for program operations in the future (absent the demonstration), CMS determined this was a reasonable basis for setting the "without waiver" cost assumptions. We further note that the carve-out would have been more costly for the federal government and would have led to

Appendix III: Comments from the Department
of Health and Human Services

GENERAL COMMENTS OF THE DEPARTMENT OF HEALTH AND HUMAN SERVICES (HHS) ON THE GOVERNMENT ACCOUNTABILITY OFFICE'S (GAO) DRAFT REPORT ENTITLED, "MEDICAID DEMONSTRATION WAIVERS: APPROVAL PROCESS RAISES CONCERNS AND LACKS TRANSPARENCY" (GAO-13-384)

fragmented care for beneficiaries. Instead, the Texas demonstration encourages integrated care and incentivizes significant delivery system reform.

In both cases, we maintain that the integrity of the budget neutrality process is intact and we stand by our calculations. As noted above, CMS has significantly strengthened the scope of accountability in Texas, as well as other demonstrations by putting conditions in place that require CMS approval before expenditures can be drawn down and by instituting robust reporting requirements to ensure effective monitoring as the demonstration projects progress.

Appendix IV: GAO Contact and Staff Acknowledgments

GAO Contact	Katherine Iritani, (202) 512-7114 or iritanik@gao.gov
Staff Acknowledgments	In addition to the contact named above, Tim Bushfield, Assistant Director; Susan Barnidge; Shirin Hormozi; Carolyn Feis Korman; Drew Long; Tom Moscovitch; Pauline Seretakis; and Hemi Tewarson made key contributions to this report.

Related GAO Products

High-Risk Series: An Update. GAO-13-283. Washington, D.C.: February 2013.

Medicaid: More Transparency of and Accountability for Supplemental Payments Are Needed. GAO-13-48. Washington, D.C.: November 26, 2012.

Medicaid: States Reported Billions More in Supplemental Payments in Recent Years. GAO-12-694. Washington, D.C.: July 20, 2012.

Medicaid Demonstration Waivers: Recent HHS Approvals Continue to Raise Cost and Oversight Concerns. GAO-08-87. Washington, D.C.: January 31, 2008.

Medicaid Demonstration Waivers: Lack of Opportunity for Public Input during Federal Approval Process Still a Concern. GAO-07-694R. Washington, D.C.: July 24, 2007.

Medicaid Waivers: HHS Approvals of Pharmacy Plus Demonstrations Continue to Raise Cost and Oversight Concerns. GAO-04-480. Washington, D.C.: June 30, 2004.

Medicaid: Improved Federal Oversight of State Financing Schemes Is Needed. GAO-04-228. Washington, D.C: February 13, 2004.

SCHIP: HHS Continues to Approve Waivers That Are Inconsistent with Program Goals. GAO-04-166R. Washington, D.C.: January 5, 2004.

Medicaid and SCHIP: Recent HHS Approvals of Demonstration Wavier Projects Raise Concerns. GAO-02-817. Washington, D.C.: July 12, 2002.

Medicaid Section 1115 Waivers: Flexible Approach to Approving Demonstrations Could Increase Federal Costs. GAO/HEHS-96-44. Washington, D.C.: November 8, 1995.

Medicaid: States Use Illusory Approaches to Shift Program Costs to Federal Government. GAO/HEHS-94-133. Washington D.C.: August 1, 1994.

GAO's Mission	The Government Accountability Office, the audit, evaluation, and investigative arm of Congress, exists to support Congress in meeting its constitutional responsibilities and to help improve the performance and accountability of the federal government for the American people. GAO examines the use of public funds; evaluates federal programs and policies; and provides analyses, recommendations, and other assistance to help Congress make informed oversight, policy, and funding decisions. GAO's commitment to good government is reflected in its core values of accountability, integrity, and reliability.
Obtaining Copies of GAO Reports and Testimony	The fastest and easiest way to obtain copies of GAO documents at no cost is through GAO's website (http://www.gao.gov). Each weekday afternoon, GAO posts on its website newly released reports, testimony, and correspondence. To have GAO e-mail you a list of newly posted products, go to http://www.gao.gov and select "E-mail Updates."
Order by Phone	The price of each GAO publication reflects GAO's actual cost of production and distribution and depends on the number of pages in the publication and whether the publication is printed in color or black and white. Pricing and ordering information is posted on GAO's website, http://www.gao.gov/ordering.htm. Place orders by calling (202) 512-6000, toll free (866) 801-7077, or TDD (202) 512-2537. Orders may be paid for using American Express, Discover Card, MasterCard, Visa, check, or money order. Call for additional information.
Connect with GAO	Connect with GAO on Facebook, Flickr, Twitter, and YouTube. Subscribe to our RSS Feeds or E-mail Updates. Listen to our Podcasts. Visit GAO on the web at www.gao.gov.
To Report Fraud, Waste, and Abuse in Federal Programs	Contact: Website: http://www.gao.gov/fraudnet/fraudnet.htm E-mail: fraudnet@gao.gov Automated answering system: (800) 424-5454 or (202) 512-7470
Congressional Relations	Katherine Siggerud, Managing Director, siggerudk@gao.gov, (202) 512-4400, U.S. Government Accountability Office, 441 G Street NW, Room 7125, Washington, DC 20548
Public Affairs	Chuck Young, Managing Director, youngc1@gao.gov, (202) 512-4800 U.S. Government Accountability Office, 441 G Street NW, Room 7149 Washington, DC 20548

Please Print on Recycled Paper.

www.ingramcontent.com/pod-product-compliance
Lightning Source LLC
Chambersburg PA
CBHW081858170526
45167CB00007B/3067